ADULT ADD
The Complete Handbook

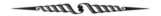

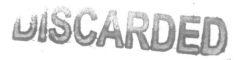

ADULT ADD
The Complete Handbook

Everything You Need to Know About
How to Cope and Live Well with
ADD/ADHD

David Sudderth, M.D.
and Joseph Kandel, M.D.

PRIMA PUBLISHING

Published by Prima Publishing, Roseville, California. Member of the Crown Publishing Group, a division of Random House, Inc.

Random House, Inc. New York, Toronto, London, Sydney, Auckland

PRIMA PUBLISHING and colophon are trademarks of Random House, Inc., registered with the United States Patent and Trademark Office.

All products mentioned in this book are trademarks of their respective companies.

The information provided in this book is not intended to be a substitute for professional or medical advice. The author and publisher specifically disclaim any liability, loss or risk, personal or otherwise, which is incurred as a result, directly or indirectly, of the use and application of any of the contents of this book.

Library of Congress Cataloging-in-Publication Data

Sudderth, David B.
Adult ADD—the complete handbook: everything you need to know about how to cope and live well with ADD/ADHD / David B. Sudderth and Joseph Kandel.
   p. cm.
Includes bibliographical references and index.
ISBN 0-7615-0796-5
   1. Attention-deficit disorder in adults—Popular works.
I. Kandel, Joseph. II. Title.
RC394.A85K36 1996
616.85'89—dc20   96-29153
                                                       CIP

01 02 03 04 HH 10 9 8 7
Printed in the United States of America

First Edition

Visit us online at www.primapublishing.com

To my sons, Alex and Felix.

—DAVID B. SUDDERTH

To Max, Hannah, and Geena—
for always keeping me focused
by seeing the world through your eyes.

—JOSEPH KANDEL

Contents

Acknowledgments

We wish to thank our staff for their constant support and patience during the writing of this manuscript. Special thanks to Kari Dibene, who keeps us organized.

Introduction

Adult attention deficit disorder is real. But there are no readily available blood tests, chemical markers, or "positive pictures"—such as an abnormal image on an MRI, CT scan, or PET scan—that a physician can use to diagnose you. (These are special studies of the brain, similar to extremely high-tech X rays.)

That is, there are no *diagnostic* tests within the price range of most patients. Yet. Researchers have found marked differences between the brains of people with ADD and people without it, and more studies are being conducted all the time. As a result, in the near future, there will almost certainly be diagnostic tests to identify ADD.

The point is, we now know for certain that ADD is a true neurobiological disorder, despite what you may have read about it being a fad or a make-believe problem. What is a neurobiological disorder? As defined in a bill filed by the U.S. House of Representatives in 1995, "neurobiological disorder" refers to one or more of these conditions: attention deficit disorder; autism or pervasive development disorder; psychotic disorders; and Tourette's syndrome.

Unfortunately, much media attention has centered on the negative when it comes to attention deficit disorder, asking such skeptical questions as, "Does it really exist, or is it just trendy to say you have it?" Positive and accurate reporting has been primarily generated by support groups and concerned physicians and mental health professionals. There are still those experts who doubt the existence of ADD. You will need to identify a physician who is a believer in and knowledgeable about ADD and chapter 5 "Where Do I Start?" offers important pointers on how to find the right expert for you.

We feel adult ADD is an extremely important topic, not only because millions of Americans have the disorder, but also because we believe it is readily amenable to a multitude of interventions. You can't make adult ADD go away completely, but there are many steps that can be taken to help someone with ADD, ranging from medication to counseling to actions the person can take herself to improve her life—whether it's as simple as taking notes when she's being given oral instructions or as high-tech as using a special watch to remind her to take the medicine or get ready for an important appointment.

This is why *Adult ADD—The Complete Handbook* not only addresses what ADD is and what causes it, but also provides practical solutions on what you can do about it. We have divided the book into three major parts. Part I includes information on the primary symptoms of attention deficit disorder, what causes it, and how physicians diagnose it. We also describe other problems that may mimic ADD or be confused with it. In addition, we include information on disorders that may coexist with attention deficit disorder.

Part II provides you with information on what to do about your ADD, including information on finding a physician, learning about medications that can help people with ADD, nonpharmacological solutions for those with ADD, and adaptive devices that can help. We also include important information on sleep disorders and health issues for ADDers and offer you advice you can implement immediately.

In part III we discuss other issues of ADD that don't fall neatly into part I or II. Women and ADD is a stand-alone chapter because for many years, most mental health professionals believed that girls and women rarely were afflicted with ADD. We now suspect that ADD in many girls and women has gone undiagnosed because they may suffer from the inattentive form of attention deficit disorder rather than the hyperactive form. Because ADD can present unique challenges to women, we address these issues in chapter 10 on women with ADD.

Why Has ADD Been Condemned?

Although adult ADD is a real disorder, some people still refuse to acknowledge it as a valid problem. One reason for this disbelief is that sometimes it takes years for the public, and even for medical practitioners, to truly accept problematic behavior as stemming from a medical disorder.

For example, in the early twentieth century, patients with a seizure disorder were often hidden away in the attic or basement by their families. Why? Because people with epilepsy were shunned by society. Likewise, patients with migraine disorders were also thought to be "out of their head" and were often ignored, not only by society as a whole, but also by the medical community.

An archaic attitude? Yes, we see that now. Seizure disorders and migraines are accepted today as neurological conditions that can be diagnosed and treated effectively.

For another example, it was not so long ago that people refused to discuss or even mention a family member with Alzheimer's disease. This was a taboo subject, and Mom or Dad were said to have "hardening of the arteries." Today we realize that this is clearly a neurodegenerative disorder and it is acceptable to talk about Alzheimer's and to actively seek treatment for it. In fact, new medications are being developed to treat this disorder even as this book is being written.

Does this mean that if you have adult ADD, it's just like having a seizure disorder or a migraine headache or Alzheimer's? Not at all, but the common denominator is that all of these problems are neurologically based disorders. They have their own unique symptoms and treatments, but they all result from a problem with the brain.

You can probably think of many other examples of illnesses that were not accepted in the past. We recall when a patient with muscle aches and pains, arthritis, joint disease, and fatigue was considered to be depressed or seeking attention. Then, when the blood test for Lyme disease (a disease caused by a tick) became known and identified, these patients were able to be diagnosed properly and treated with medications. Many improved dramatically. (In fact, some people who are diagnosed with ADD actually have Lyme disease! See chapter 4, on differential diagnosis.)

Patients who suffer from attention deficit disorder should not be relegated to a second-class position. Nor should they be given short shrift by the health care community for seeking medical attention and intervention.

Not Just for Kids Anymore

Another very important point to keep in mind is that for many years ADD was considered to be only a disorder of childhood. Once a person with ADD reached adolescence, the medications were usually discontinued because physicians believed that ADD was something you "grew out of." Despite impassioned pleas by some parents of teenagers, the medical community turned its back on teens with ADD. And adults? Forget it. It was presumed that teenagers or adults who sought medications for ADD were really after stimulating drugs to give them feelings of euphoria, an artificial "high." (Actually, stimulant medications do not have such an effect on people with ADD.)

We now know that anywhere from 20 to 35 percent or more of the children diagnosed with ADD will continue into adulthood with some manifestation of their disorder. Add to that the many adults who were NOT diagnosed with ADD as children, even though they did have this disorder. The numbers grow.

While it is true that hyperactivity routinely improves with adolescence and young adulthood, the impulsivity, inattention, and disorganization of thought often carry through into adulthood and impose a dramatic impact on a sufferer's life.

How many adults have ADD? Statistics indicate that from one to three percent of the adult population may have some form of ADHD. However, longitudinal (long-term) studies are few in this dramatically changing field, and we are really at the infancy, or possibly toddlerhood, of understanding this relatively newly acknowledged disorder of adults.

About the Authors

We are board-certified neurologists who treat attention deficit disorder in children and adults. We are also expert in treating many other diseases, some of which can mimic ADD.

To research our book, we relied on journal articles and books, as well as our own experience. But to expand even further, we also surveyed people with ADD on the Internet and also on the ADD Forum of CompuServe. These individuals provided some powerful anecdotes and insights that we feel will help our readers.

Overview of the Book

We cover many critical issues in this book, issues that affect you and your family. In fact, the family of the ADD individual is usually profoundly affected, so we include information not only on the problem areas but also on empowering solutions that individuals can try.

In chapter 1, describing what ADD is and what it is not, we discuss why it is important to identify it as a true neurological illness, and how this acknowledgment can provide an explanation to an otherwise hectic and chaotic life and lifestyle. The American Psychiatric Association, through the *Diagnostic and Statistical Manual IV,* has outlined very specific criteria for ADD. We explain why we feel that individuals with ADD are actually *underdiagnosed,* with those who are currently diagnosed representing the tip of the iceberg.

Diagnosing ADD can be much more difficult than you might expect, even for an experienced medical doctor or psychologist. If you remember back to elementary school, when there was always one child having a sign placed on his back that said "kick me"—a sign that all the other children could see but the child wearing it could not—individuals with ADD sometimes cannot identify or comprehend their own disorder.

As a result, we have included in appendix IV a sample questionnaire that should help determine whether you have ADD. This could be an important tool to review with your physician and may actually be very helpful in further clarifying your thinking on this disorder.

Because there are often additional illnesses (called "comorbidity") associated with ADHD, we discuss various psychological and psychiatric disorders, such as major depression, addictive personality, and substance abuse, to help you understand why it is so difficult for physicians, as well as for the general public, to make an accurate diagnosis.

Possibly one of the most helpful sections in this book is chapter 9 about adaptive devices, ranging from low technology all the way to very sophisticated instruments. These are tools that can significantly help an individual with an unstructured and disorganized lifestyle become more productive, structured, and successful in achieving specific goals. It is important to understand that this topic is changing dramatically, and in chapter 9 we outline how the reader can keep up with all these current and exciting changes.

We also discuss specific problems that ADDers may have, such as difficulties with sleep and what you can do if you are one of many ADD insomniacs. And we talk about the value of exercise in helping the person with ADD to not only improve health but to better focus his life.

What about medications? If you have suffered with ADHD, it is absolutely impossible for you to have missed the raging firestorm over the use of central nervous system stimulants such as Ritalin or Dexedrine. Are people overtreated? Are people overdiagnosed? We will answer these questions. We will state here, however, that in many cases, people with ADHD who are on appropriate medications have a very positive and favorable response.

Just as we would not want our patients with diabetes or hypertension to be overly distressed about becoming "hooked" on their diabetes medicine or blood pressure medicines, once the diagnosis for ADD is accurately and correctly made, we don't harp on the issue of chemical addiction. We do, however, discuss the issue of habituation and the need for ongoing medication therapy versus switching around to various modalities of treatment. We explain when treatment can be successfully tapered and also cover some of the warning signs to watch for when medications are changed.

While we are actively practicing physicians and are traditional in terms of patient management, we also realize there is a wide spectrum of treatment, including nontraditional therapies, drugs, and behavior-adaptive techniques. The importance of psychological counseling cannot be ignored, so we discuss why and how therapy can be very helpful to the person with ADD.

In addition, ADHD has a significant impact in the workplace, probably costing millions of dollars. We discuss the impact of ADD as a disabling condition, both to the individual employer and to coworkers, as well as to society as a whole. The Americans with Disabilities Act (ADA) includes ADD as a disability, and thus workers can request work accommodations.

Above all, *Adult ADD—The Complete Handbook* is a self-help guide to provide education, information, and hope. As with most other illnesses, the more you learn about the disease, the better prepared you are not only to face family and friends, but also to become a better patient in the doctor-patient relationship. We discuss this issue in chapter 5, on starting out and learning how to begin your diagnostic health care journey toward improvement in your ADHD.

Our primary goal is that this book will offer you an explanation and understanding of your current illness, as well as workable solutions you can try out. Keep in mind, however, that we don't see ADD as an excuse. Just as an individual suffering from blood pressure or diabetes does not have any kind of "permission" to behave improperly, neither do individuals with ADD gain an excuse for their behavior. Rather, the disorder should be construed as a framework for your actions and behaviors, your disorganization and your interactions with peers, family, friends, and coworkers.

Knowledge is power. We have been told repeatedly by our grateful patients that just knowing there is a rational, medical explanation for their constant procrastination, disorganization, and, at times, social disabilities, has helped them devise strategies to change these behaviors, improve their interactions, and organize themselves in a way to produce a positive change. We have heard repeatedly, "Knowing I wasn't crazy made all the difference and really helped me get my life under control." We hope this book will do the same for you.

ADULT ADD
The Complete Handbook

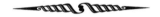

Identifying the Problem

1

What Is ADD?

⟨decorative ornament⟩

Attention deficit disorder is a pervasive symptom complex involving inattention, impulsivity, distractibility, and hyperactivity. A number of other behavior characteristics are frequently seen in individuals suffering from this illness and will be discussed at length in chapter 3. In this chapter we will provide a detailed description of ADD's characteristics. (And in chapter 4, on differential diagnosis, we'll show you what ADD is *not.*) We will also speculate on why another neurological disorder, Alzheimer's disease, has been widely accepted while ADD, equally valid in a scientific sense, has been widely derided by the press and even by physicians.

Historical Perspectives

In 1907, an obscure European physician named Alois Alzheimer described a case of a deceased 51-year-old woman who had developed difficulty with memory, language, and paranoid delusions during her later years. The autopsy on this woman demonstrated some peculiar, previously undescribed microscopic changes in the appearance of the woman's brain when examined under a light microscope. These changes, tangles of abnormally accumulated material, ultimately formed the basis for the diagnosis of what is known today as Alzheimer's disease. Prior to 1960, probably fewer than a hundred cases of this illness were reported in world literature. But by the mid 1990s, this disease is considered to be the fourth most common cause of death in the United States. Persons and families afflicted with this progressive, debilitating illness are viewed with the greatest sympathy by society. Alzheimer is now a household name.

Only five years before Alzheimer's report, another new disease hit the medical press. In 1902, Dr. George Still reported on a behavioral syndrome in children in the esteemed British medical journal *Lancet.* Still described the behavior of the children he observed in such terms as "abnormal deficits in moral control," "wanton mischievousness" and "destructiveness." (Today we would probably subdivide the group of children reported by Still as children with ADD, conduct disorder (CD), and oppositional defiant disorder (ODD). While one rarely encounters the term "wanton mischievousness" in the media today, there are plenty of doubts and negative labels conveyed by reporters on ADD. Interestingly, this same doubt is virtually nonexistent when the same reporters write about Alzheimer's disease.

Why victims of these two diseases are treated in such a dissimilar manner is one of the many mysteries surrounding attention deficit disorder, which rests on as firm a scientific basis as does Alzheimer's disease.

First Treatment of ADD

The first report of effective pharmacological treatment of ADD was published in 1937 by C. Bradley, who described a group of children, ages five to thirteen, who demonstrated more organized behavior when given oral amphetamine. This medication was known to have high abuse potential among adults, who had a markedly different response to the medication, i.e., euphoric state, craving, etc. (It's important to note that adults with ADD do not experience feelings of euphoria and craving when they take amphetamines or other medications for ADD.)

At that time, it was a controversial practice to give this medication to children, when it clearly had a highly addicting effect on many people; the debate for and against the use of such stimulant medications persists to this day. The fearsome specter of a harsh and demanding society forcing small children to consume large amounts of potentially addictive or otherwise harmful medications frightened those who did not understand the positive impact of stimulants on those who need them.

Later, methylphenidate (Ritalin) became available as a treatment for ADD, as did the medication pemoline (Cylert). Many subsequent controlled studies have demonstrated that these medications are quite effective in providing symptomatic relief from the various troubling behavioral aspects of ADD.

Over the last three decades, various journal articles have suggested that some of the symptoms seen in children with attention deficit disorder persist well into adulthood. Yet it was not until 1978, in Scottsdale, Arizona, that a conference on the subject was held—a conference that attracted very little attention. Then, in the early 1980s, increasing numbers of reports in the press indicated that adult ADD was actually a genuine diagnostic entity, and in 1989 an adult ADD clinic was opened at Wayne State University in Detroit.

Seemingly overnight, adult ADD support groups appeared in many states, newsletters directed at adults with ADD began to circulate, and support groups such as the very popular CH.A.D.D. (Children and Adults with Attention Deficit Disorder) were founded.

In 1990, Dr. Alan J. Zametkin and his colleagues published an article in the prestigious *New England Journal of Medicine* that identified a metabolic defect in adults with attention deficit disorder. This article detailed a controlled study in which the brain's ability to utilize glucose was impaired in a person with attention deficit disorder but was normal in people without ADD. This article legitimized attention deficit disorder as a formal diagnostic entity.

Since then, many articles about attention deficit disorder in adults have been published, and in 1992 psychologist Lynn Weiss published *Attention Deficit Disorder in Adults,* the first book on ADD in adults for nonprofessional readers.[1] After the publication of Weiss's book, a virtual explosion of information and interest in ADD among children and adults has dominated the print and broadcast media, but much of the media attention has been negative.

Why Was ADD Ignored for So Long?

Physicians have a long history of assuring parents that various problems will be "outgrown" as the patient approaches adulthood, and ADD was no exception. Although it is true that most children do typically outgrow some conditions such as bedwetting and petit mal seizures, other disease states are not outgrown. Another explanation for this delay in the recognition of ADD is unquestionably related to adaptation and compensation by the patient. Adult attention deficit disorder patients frequently have developed various strategies for dealing with their problems which enable them to support themselves and "get by."

Also, many other conditions are frequently seen in patients with ADD or may be a consequence of the ADD. As a result, this other condition may dominate the patient's overall disability while the ADD component is less obvious to the

---

1. Lynn Weiss, *Attention Deficit Disorder in Adults: Practical Help for Suffers and Their Spouses.* (Dallas: Taylor, 1992.)

treating physician. Thus, if a person was depressed and also had ADD, it was more likely that the depression would be diagnosed rather than the ADD.

Furthermore, medical knowledge races ahead at atomic velocities while medical practice proceeds in accordance with its own internal pocket watch.

Another relevant factor is that an increasingly involved and educated lay public has largely imposed its own time-keeping strategies on doctors, often pressuring them into taking positions and responding faster with regard to accepting an illness than with the wait-and-see positions many doctors have taken in the past.

ADD: What's in a Name?

Attention deficit disorder has gone through various terminology rites of passage before reaching its current nomenclature. The term *minimal brain damage/dysfunction* (MBD) was current at one point, as was *hyperkinetic reaction of childhood* (HRC). *Attention deficit disorder* (ADD) and *attention deficit hyperactivity disorder* (ADHD) are the terms used by most authorities today. This terminology is far from perfect, and we predict that these names will be replaced in the near future, as a more precise understanding of this disorder is achieved and its various subgroups are identified.

In this book, we will use the terms *attention deficit disorder* and ADD rather than ADHD because many of our readers will have ADD but will not experience hyperactivity as a major problem—or a problem at all.

Primary Symptoms of ADD

Below we list and briefly describe the most commonly experienced primary symptoms of attention deficit disorder. If you don't see yourself in all of these, understand that each person with ADD is different and exhibits different symptoms and different degrees of symptoms (mild, moderate, and severe). Also, the problems that one person has may be no obstacle for another person with ADD. Although symptoms among people with ADD vary, most exhibit the symptoms of impulsivity and inattention, while others exhibit hyperactivity. We'll discuss these symptoms and others in this section.

Impulsivity

Impulsivity, or impulsiveness, appears to be one of the features of ADD which changes very little throughout the course of an ADDer's life. This uncritical, seemingly reflexive tendency to respond to various external stimuli can be the most disabling and even dangerous feature of adult attention deficit disorder.

Impulsiveness in children is often overlooked by adults and is sometimes even viewed as "cute." In the adult world, however, this type of behavior is poorly tolerated and rarely goes unpunished. Impulsive behavior can ruin you financially, cause you to lose your job and your family, or even saddle you with a fatal sexually transmitted disease.

One of our patients, Steven J., reported some difficulties at work, which allowed him the "privilege" of changing jobs twenty times in one year. (Note: all names have been changed in our anecdotes about people with ADD.)

The longest job I've ever had lasted six months and I would have been fired long before that if people knew what I was actually doing. I tend to annoy people immensely by blurting out whatever comes into my mind and constantly interrupting people around me. My boss would give me one job but I would get bogged down in one part of the task or altogether start on something new. Every time I began a new job I thought of ten other things that I should be doing at the same time. This often led to my not being able to accomplish

the task set before me during the course of the day,
leaving me with ambitious but totally unrealistic plans
of finishing at home.
*   Invariably I would go home, grab something to eat,*
check my mail, "relax on the computer," make a few
phone calls, and by then it was midnight and I was too
tired to even think about the work, which, by the way, I
had left in my car. Although I replayed this script over
and over again, I was equally surprised every time. The
next day I would take my unfinished work back into the
office, make my excuses and do it all over again.

Steven brings up several difficult issues facing the ADDer, including verbal "impetuosity." A person with ADD is faced with an urgent need to express ideas "before they get away" from him. He (and others like him) seems to lack mental filing cabinets where information can be stored and retrieved at will. This unquestionably is one reason an ADDer is pressured to relieve himself of his thoughts and ideas.

As noted elsewhere in this book, individuals with ADD often have unique insights and creative impulses that "evaporate" if not mediated to other individuals, written down, or otherwise put on "hard copy." The concept of "inspiration preservation," our phrase for saving your creative ideas, will be discussed elsewhere in this book, and we'll suggest various strategies to avoid losing creative ideas. (See chapter 8 and 9 for more information.)

Individuals with ADD can be virtual "verbal howitzers" firing in a semirandom, absolutely automatic manner at anyone, hostile and friendly. Spouses and children are often the objects of ill-conceived remarks that are generated and executed before the ADDer has really contemplated the consequences of these remarks. Close friends and family members of individuals with this particularly annoying tendency can learn to accept this to a certain degree. Spouses often report being socially embarrassed by the involuntary verbal outbursts of someone with this disorder. The other side of this coin is that individuals with ADD are often very quick with witty repartee or anecdotes.

ADD-related impulsivity can also lead to financial catastrophes.

We met Eric G. at the referral of his wife, who had attended the diagnostic interviews with the couple's son who also had ADD. [Often, parents discover that they have ADD after their own children are diagnosed.] Eric presented a fairly typical history of attention deficit disorder. He had scored highly on the mathematic portion of his SAT but had flunked out of college calculus. He presented other examples of "flashes of brilliance" in his past, but more often he functioned at a level well below his abilities.

As a young man, Eric had dropped out of college and taken a job in a hardware store. He was well liked by his coworkers, who covered for him frequently when his impulsivity and other characteristics of ADD got him into trouble.

Eric had resolved with his wife's help to open a small store. The couple had outlined a five-year plan, involving savings, part-time jobs, etc., which would enable them to save enough to finance their dream. But every time the family saved up a few thousand dollars, Eric would make a major purchase without consulting his spouse. He'd bought boats, paid for vacations he planned without discussing it with his wife, and committed other acts of financial incontinence, thus rendering the couples dreams unattainable.

Said Eric, "I don't know why she stays with me. If impulse purchases were tattoos I would be 'butterfly man.'"

Through counseling and the adoption of various strategies as well as medication therapy, Eric has greatly improved in controlling his impulsivity. However, he still works for someone else.

Sexuality

The sexual arena is another hostile environment for the impulsive. People who engage in sexual practices without care or considering the possible consequences of unwanted pregnancies or broken marriages are taking a great risk. Impulsive people, however, may take such risks. And of course the biggest risk to unprotected sex is the scourge of our time, HIV infection.

Hyperactivity

One feature of ADD that often is said to improve with age is hyperactivity. It always starts in childhood, but only on rare occasions does it get worse in adulthood. The reason for the apparent improvement of hyperactivity in adults may be related to learned behavior and an increased ability to control actions. This doesn't mean that the hyperactivity goes away—although it can. More likely, the adult has learned better ways to cope with it.

While a child may jump up and down in a chair, dart from room to room, or move objects about in a room, the adult will tend to have less obtrusive behavior such as finger tapping, frequent shifting while seated, and frequent readjustment of the arms and legs. Rapid and seemingly incessant speech is also another manifestation of this hyperactive tendency.

Said John B., "My mind is constantly going and I wear some folks out. I have boundless energy and swarms of ideas, but I have finally found my niche in life." (He is a freelance photographer, with constant changes of his environment.)

Tim L. is a police officer with ADD. He says, "I am always kidded with because I do everything fast. I have to always be doing something. I find it almost impossible to hand-write reports; everything must be typed because I can do it faster that way."

Hyperactivity is often not an endearing quality. Karen S. relates,

I've certainly been no stranger to the job market. I've had any number of jobs. At one point I took a job for a floor covering company which had many employees, including a large sales force. I really liked my boss, who seemed to have some understanding of my various problems, as did many of the coworkers. However, my fidgetiness and inability to stay at my post led to an essentially intolerable situation for my coworkers.

My boss had noticed that I had dealt fairly with customers and suggested that maybe I should be relocated to the sales force. My new job as a salesperson proved advantageous for all. I could get out of the office where I would not annoy or distract the other staff and so on. Calling on customers, exchanging small talk, and presenting new ideas to the buyers has been something that I have enjoyed. I have made many innovations in our company's approach to customers, which have also been adopted by other salespersons. My boss is happy, my coworkers are happy and so are my customers. I'm still hyper and I can still be irritating, but for the first time I feel that I have some job security.

Hyperactivity can be a real burden for the ADDer as well as for others in her life. Interpersonal relationships often are put to the test by this particular trait. One person may like to engage in open-ended conversations, while the hyperactive person with ADD may find long discussions intolerable. This type of dilemma can lead to great dissatisfaction on both parts and even to failed relationships.

Inattention

At the core of any discussion of this disorder is, of course, attention itself. Individuals suffering from attention deficit disorder actually appear to be able to attain a normal level of attention at least periodically. What seems to happen is that they are unable to maintain their attention level willfully for satisfying periods of time. An analogy would be the case of petit mal seizures, a type of epilepsy primarily affecting young persons. In this disorder, the patient will temporarily lose consciousness but maintain body control, posture, etc. The person has essentially no recall of the brief period of time he is "away."

While the ADDer does not actually lose consciousness, there is a gap in which sensory input is essentially lost. One patient told us: "This is what I envy most about 'normies.' They seem to own their attention. I don't own mine but occasionally I get to borrow it." These symptoms lead to the person with ADD being called "space cadet," "airhead," and other derogatory epithets. This disordered attention maintenance can lead to pervasively impaired functioning in essentially all aspects of daily living.

In our high-tech culture, in which education is highly valued, inattentiveness can be a serious liability. One college student told us that it was pointless to go to lectures.

> *Within five minutes I would be entranced in a multilayered daydream with no apparent beginning or end. Occasionally I would surface for air but quickly return back to my mind-wandering. My attention is usually something like the ocean ebbing in and out at the beach. Less often it's like a tidal wave. There is no in between.*

The attention impairment can also be compared to a random, sensory filter that deprives the person with ADD of verbal or written information, regardless of its importance. Besides being a major handicap in the classroom, it can be almost paralyzing for the ADDer who occasionally is called upon to follow verbal directions. Says Harry B.,

> *I had a very brief career as a pizza deliverer. Actually, I was able to keep the job only for two days. Every time I*

was given a pizza, I was also given detailed verbal instructions on finding the delivery site. Usually I write this type of information down but did not want to call attention to myself. The cars were equipped with radios and it would usually take me three or four calls back to the restaurant before I would finally get to my destination with a very cold pizza. This problem has caused irritation in some of my other jobs but this was unquestionably the worst example.

This problem of "zoning out" can be particularly irritating in personal relationships. Conducting routine family life requires close cooperation and communication between the two partners and can involve very lengthy discussions. Despite the ADDer's best attention, he frequently falls short of the mark. One person explained, "my wife always knows when she's losing me. It used to drive her crazy. Now she has learned to "retrieve the lost space shuttle," as she calls it, by saying something to grab my attention or by touching me."

Said another man with ADD,

None of my girlfriends has had ADD. Often they felt that I didn't care about them because I would become distracted and inattentive. My priorities are often out of whack, so I am often late for everything. They believed that I didn't have enough respect for them to be on time. Before I found out about ADD, I couldn't understand why I did these things to them when I knew in my heart that I really cared for them and that my actions were not motivated by malice.

Sometimes the inattentiveness can lead to amusing results. Mary L. says she'd drive to the supermarket at 2 A.M. to get milk for breakfast, and find herself at work instead—she'd automatically driven there without thinking.

Difficulties with maintaining attention over a prolonged period of time can be very disabling when it comes to completing tasks. The brain of a person with ADD can be likened to the navigational system in a plane. When an airplane begins its journey, it heads roughly toward its destination. Flight navigation updates enable a fairly straight trajectory throughout the trip. But for the ADDer, occasionally these course updates never reach the navigation instrument, thus leading the person to stray frequently off target—although he usually does arrive eventually. This failure leads to an enormous amount of wasted effort and time.

Another very problematic feature of ADD which is also related to inattention is that there are great variations from day to day in the person's attention span. One day, a task can be performed well, and thus others believe it has been mastered. But perhaps the next day, the task is done poorly or forgotten, thus leading others without ADD to think the person is not really trying. In fact, if you have ADD, you could be trying even harder on the second day, but your innate attention problem is holding you back.

Consider an analogy with another neurologic disease, Parkinson's disease. Individuals suffering from this disorder experience difficulty with initiating motion, balance, and various other motor functions. Yet it is well known that individuals with severe Parkinson's disease and seriously impaired functioning level can rise above their illness for brief periods of time—usually related to such emergencies as a fire or endangerment of life. We can relate this experience to what Frank B. told us.

I had a fairly incredible academic career. I would usually be at the top of the class when it came to aptitude tests. I always found these fairly interesting and there was really no way to prepare for them. However, for the routine examinations in which we were usually warned repeatedly ahead of time, I would typically be at the bottom when the scores were handed out.

One teacher, who had taken a special interest in my performance, often chastised me because of the

*unevenness in my performance. She often made me feel
I was being punished for my successes. She even went
so far at one point as to say, "Frank, you're the smartest
and the dumbest kid in the class."*

This paralyzing impairment in attention maintenance may lead to diminished performance in academics, personal relationships, workplace efficiency, and other areas of life. The problem can render the ADDer a hostage to the present and can also lead to other serious problems that may be worse than the attention deficit disorder itself, such as depression, loss of self-esteem, lack of financial independence, drug use, and multiple failed relationships.

I'll Think About That Tomorrow: Procrastination

Scarlett O'Hara, heroine of *Gone with the Wind,* delayed important decisions when she faced a crisis. "After all, tomorrow is another day." But many people with ADD procrastinate as a way of life, and this can generate plenty of problems. Many of our patients have told us about their extreme difficulty with deadlines and timetables, and report that they suffer from chronic tardiness.

Although procrastination is one of the most troublesome characteristics of attention deficit disorder, we find that our patients who worry about this problem are usually attending to too many objects. They are easily distracted and consequently they become frequently bored with routine activities, and so ignore the mundane, day-to-day matters that must be attended to. We try to help them prioritize what they need to do and focus on the most important issues and tasks.

Fortunately, there are medications and strategies that people with ADD can use to deal with the symptoms we've just described. We discuss a range of solutions in Part II.

2

Causes of ADD

―――◦ᚱᚱᚱᚱᚱ ⸘ ᚱᚱᚱᚱᚱᚱ◦―――

"Men ought to know that from the brain, and from the brain only, arise our pleasures, joys, laughter and gests, as well as our sorrows, pains, griefs and tears. . . . It is the same thing which makes us mad or delirious, inspires us with dread and fear, whether by night or by day, brings sleepiness, inopportune mistakes, aimless anxieties, absentmindedness and acts that are contrary to habit." —*Hippocrates*

In this chapter, we focus on what researchers and physicians know about this brain disorder. The information provided in this chapter presents scientific research and evidence for the existence of ADD.

People with ADD can develop a good mastery and understanding of their illness, and clearly have a vested interest in devoting the time and effort to doing so. For these reasons, we feel it's important to begin with a clear presentation of physiologic processes believed to be at work in ADD. This is based on our firm belief that when you invest the time to learn about your illness and are willing to share the responsibility with your physicians, then you will ultimately get the best care. This is true of migraine and back pain (on which we have published books), and certainly is also true for ADD.

First, let's start with some basic anatomical information about that most important organ—your brain.

The Brain and Central Nervous System

Your brain is an extremely active organ with constant electrical impulses traveling back and forth and special chemicals called neurotransmitters that aid (or impair) the transmission of these impulses. The problem for the person with ADD may be that the brain may have some minor damage to a specific area, such as the frontal lobe. Or the biochemicals may be insufficient to do a good job. There are a variety of things that can go awry, and we will talk about several in our section on possible causes of ADD, later in this chapter. First, however, let's look at some basic anatomy.

The central nervous system consists of two primary parts: the brain and the spinal cord. Various nerves exit their long bony encasement from the spinal cord and the brain and are found in different parts of the body. These nerves allow us to move and perceive our surroundings through sensory mechanisms. Our ability to move, see, hear, make love, feel the texture of cloth—as well as manage more complex processes such as thinking, feeling, and reasoning—the ability to perform these daily tasks depends entirely upon one nerve cell's ability to communicate with another nerve cell.

Like copper wires, neurons (nerve cells) conduct electrical energy from one portion of the nerve cell to the other. Actual copper wires can be connected by splicing or by connecting two wires to a switch. But one neuron cannot affect the behavior or activity of another neuron by direct conduction of an electrical impulse. This means you can't splice neurons. (At least, not yet.)

Between any two nerves is a small space called the *synaptic cleft*. This indirect connection between portions of two adjacent, related nerve cells is called a *synapse*. It is in this microscopic arena that numerous molecular titans participate in a complex struggle that ultimately determines the course of human behavior. The portion of the "incoming" neuron is called the *presynaptic membrane* while the portion of the "outgoing" neuron is called the *postsynaptic membrane.*

The outcome of this connection occurring in the synaptic cleft can result in activation, which means the initiating of the conduction of a nerve impulse facilitation. Or it can result in reduction in the likelihood of the nerve conducting an impulse(inhibition).

Neurotransmitters and Neuroreceptors

Neurotransmitters are chemical messengers released from nerve endings and they have a profound effect on human behavior. The main transmitters that we will discuss are dopamine, norepinephrine, and serotonin. There are many other neurotransmitters but for our purposes, these three are the main ones. We'll have more to say on neurotransmitters later in this chapter.

Michael Jordan and Neurons

Let's look at the action of neurotransmitters and neuroreceptors, using an analogy of a basketball game. Compare the action of Michael Jordan, the famous basketball player, to the action of a nerve. Let's say that Jordan grabs a basketball, jumps in the air and slam-dunks the ball (neurotransmitter) into the hoop receptor. Compare this to the neurotransmitter activating the postsynaptic neuron—the scoreboard. But remember, winning or losing the game is not decided by this one occurrence. If, however, Jordan or his teammates place the basketball in the hoop enough times during the course of the game, then the game is won by the Chicago Bulls. And if the postsynaptic neuron is stimulated enough times, then a new electrical impulse is generated.

Keep in mind if Jordan threw another type of ball in the hoop, such as a baseball, it would have no effect on the scoreboard. In the same way, a neuroreceptor will only respond to a very specific neurotransmitter. No substitutions are allowed. Imagine for a moment what it would be like if the air of the stadium were suddenly filled with scores of bowling balls. In that case, even Michael Jordan would have difficulty finding the basket. The scoring procedure is not always as easy as Michael Jordan would make it appear. For example, the shot can be blocked by an opposing player. Following our analogy, the blocking of a neurotransmitter by another molecule can impair the coupling of the neurotransmitter to the receptor molecule.

Localization of Brain Function

Continuing our analogy, other ballgames are being played at all times—let's say football, baseball, and golf. Now, of course, these games are not played on the same field. They are localized to their own specific region or field. This brings us to the important neurologic concept of *localization.*

Many credit this early concept of localization to the French scientist Joseph Gall, who suggested that the various functions, such as the ability to move, speak, and perform other activities, related directly to specific areas of the brain. This led to scientists deciding to study people with neurologic problems, by postmortem examinations of their brains.

The French neurologist Paul Broca observed a patient for many years, whose only utterance was "pa-pa." Upon the death of this individual, Dr. Broca examined the patient's brain and found an area of destruction in the left side of the brain. Even to this day, this area of the brain, "Broca's" area, is discussed by clinicians as the language center.

Of course, the production of language is infinitely more complex than originally assumed; however, the principle of location still applies to the organizational scheme of the brain of any advanced species.

Frontal Lobes of the Brain

Now let's look at a very important part of the brain, the frontal lobes. They are quite huge in the human brain, occupying approximately one half of the cerebrum—the portion of the brain above the brainstem. The posterior portion of the frontal lobe is involved with language, motor activities, and sensation. The anterior portion of the frontal lobe is intimately related to features of behavior which are uniquely human, such as sequencing, drive, and an executive control. Executive control is one area which is very problematic for the person with ADD.

Sequencing, Drive, and Executive Control

Sequencing ability, also known as *working memory,* is the ability to handle information in a stepwise manner, despite distractions. The doctor tests the ability to sequence by having the patient reproduce finger tapping rhythms or copy a series of letters provided by the examiner or perform other sequential tasks.

Drive refers to a person's ability to accomplish the tasks at hand. Injury to the frontal lobes can cause apathy and lack of motivation. Frontal lobe injury can also lead to a state of mental and physical agitation, particularly when the middle portions of the frontal lobe are affected.

Executive control is more difficult to observe clinically. Executive control refers largely to skills related to social appropriateness. Loss of executive control leads to a release of behaviors that are viewed in the adult world as primitive or ill-conceived. Dysfunction in this feature of control can lead to an awkward degree of frankness (blurting out comments that may offend), impulsivity, distractibility, and difficulty with task completion. Sound like anyone we know? Here's where the ADD comes in.

> *"Sometimes I feel like I should read myself my rights before I speak!" said Carol L. "You know, you have the right to remain silent, anything you say can be used against you. Maybe people who don't have ADD have that inner sense—but I don't! From my brain to your ears, and it's gotten me into trouble sometimes."*

Scientists are interested in this problem as well as the other dysfunctions associated with ADD, and fortunately, researchers in the medical field have made enormous progress in studying the frontal lobes as well as the brain in general. Anatomic imaging studies such as magnetic resonance imaging (MRI) as well as computerized tomography (CT scan) provide us with very accurate images of the brain's appearance.

In addition, beyond studying the brain in an anatomic sense, exciting new technologies have also become available to the modern researcher in the form of functional imaging tests, such as positron emission tomography (PET) and single photon emission computer tomography (SPECT) scans.

The Limbic System

Aside from the more advanced portions of the brain, such as the frontal lobes, other specialized groups of neurons exist in the deeper and more primitive sections. One of these regions is the limbic system. The limbic system appears to be the center of emotion. It is through the function of this complex network of neurons that pleasure, fear, and other emotions are mediated. The activity of the limbic system, well-connected to the frontal lobes, is a major player in the dopamine game (which we'll describe in more detail later in this chapter).

Now you have some basic information about your brain and how it works, and we can move on to theories of what actually causes attention deficit disorder.

Theories of What Causes ADD

At this point, we will consider various explanations for what actually causes people to have attention deficit disorder. We'll describe five different theories that purport to explain what causes this disorder, and will briefly mention other theories that scientists believe may cause or affect ADD. Keep in mind, however, that there is no perfect explanation for exactly what is happening in the brain of a person experiencing this disorder. We also anticipate that other theories will be developed over the next few years. In addition, we expect that existing theories to explain ADD will become more refined as functional imaging tests (such as MRIs and PET scans) are used even more efficiently and more frequently than now and as new and better tools and techniques are developed.

We've seen this with many other neurologic conditions, such as stroke, epilepsy, migraine, dementia, and other symptom complexes. They were initially diagnosed clinically by a physician, based on a typical symptom complex. Later, MRI and other tools provided a backup (or refuting) of the doctor's diagnosis.

Many theorists also believe that ADD can be explained as a genetic predisposition that a person inherits. These various theories are not mutually exclusive and there are overlappings. For example, it is possible to believe that ADD has a genetic basis and that it is also a biochemical disorder. In this case, the biochemical disorder could have been inherited.

We believe that human behavior is a very complex phenomenon and can only be meaningfully discussed in the context of an interplay between genetic/biochemical factors and interaction with the environment. For example, a person could inherit a genetic predisposition to becoming an alcoholic. But if he never consumes alcohol, then he will not become an alcoholic—thus environment has a direct impact on behavior.

The Catecholamine Theory

We discussed neurotransmitters earlier in this chapter. Neurotransmitters are biochemicals that are released by one nerve cell to influence a second nerve cell, either in an inhibitory or stimulating manner. There are at least thirty known or suspected chemicals that act as neurotransmitters. *Dopamine, norepinephrine,* and *serotonin* belong to the group of neurotransmitters called *catecholamines.* These neurotransmitters are intimately involved in such complex behavioral phenomena as depression, pain, anxiety, sleep, attention, alertness, as well as aggression. They tend to be localized in various pathways or systems.

In one interesting study reported in 1995, three groups of children were studied to see if their urinary catecholamines were different. One group was comprised of "pure" attention deficit children, another group was made up of children with ADD who were also diagnosed with anxiety disorder, and the third group was made up of normal children.

Each group was given tasks to perform, and then their excretions of epinephrine, norepinephrine, and other substances were measured. The children in the two ADD groups excreted more normetanephrine, which is a part of norepinephrine. Comparing the two ADD groups, researchers found that the anxious children with ADD excreted more epinephrine than did the ADD children without anxiety. This test showed clearly different chemical responses between children with and without ADD, more evidence that ADD is real.

Dopamine is another substance that may be involved with ADD. Responses to amphetamine or cocaine appear to increase the amount of dopamine in the synaptic cleft. This may be why individuals with ADD who use cocaine do not report the euphoric high that others say they experience. Instead, they say that cocaine makes them feel normal. (We would much prefer that they use a lawful medication prescribed by a physician.)

Medications such as reserpine reduce the available dopamine in the synaptic cleft. Reserpine has been used in the past for individuals with severe high blood pressure, but is used rarely today, primarily because of its tendency to cause severe depression and even suicide.

Chemicals in living tissue are constantly being produced, transported, stored, and broken down. If dopamine were involved in attention deficit disorder, then it would be reasonable to think that the breakdown products of dopamine would be abnormally low in the cerebral spinal fluid (CSF), the fluid surrounding the brain. Studies have revealed that this does happen.

One study reported by Shaywitz, et al., demonstrated that children with attention deficit disorder tended to have lower levels of the breakdown products of dopamine in their cerebral spinal fluid than normal controls.

Another interesting study is the one reported by Reimherr, et al. In this powerful study, fifteen adults with attention deficit disorder and hyperactivity, and thirteen adults who did not have ADD, were tested with regard to cerebrospinal fluid waste products, both before and after treatment with methylphenidate. (Methylphenidate is the active ingredient of Ritalin, which is often used to treat ADD.)

Eleven of the ADD subjects improved considerably after taking the methylphenidate, while four got worse or showed little improvement. Those who responded to methylphenidate tended to have lower levels of dopamine-related waste products, while those who did not respond had higher amounts of waste products of dopamine. These two studies provide a very powerful argument supporting the theory that attention deficit disorder is related to an impaired function of the dopamine system.

Other studies have involved the administration of large amounts of dopamine precursor markers. These are markers that ultimately are chemically transformed to dopamine. One of these, tyrosine, was found to be fairly effective in alleviating many of the symptoms of attention deficit disorder. However, the effects were short-lived.

Other research was based on the observation that dopamine concentration in the synaptic cleft can be increased by slowing down the rate at which dopamine is degraded. Children with ADD who were given Eldepryl and Pargyline demonstrated some improvement, but some experienced unpleasant side effects, particularly with Eldepryl. (See chapter 6 on medications for ADD.)

The Theory of Frontal Lobe Failure

An increasing volume of evidence now implicates frontal lobe function impairment as the primary area of malfunction in attention deficit disorder. When our senses of touch, sight, hearing, taste, and smell are stimulated, impulses travel from the skin, eyes, and ears to specific areas in the cerebral cortex. (The *cerebral cortex* is the multilayered system of neurons on the surface of the brain.) These impulses are ultimately relayed to neurons lying deep within the limbic system, which was described earlier in the chapter.

The limbic system then compares the sensory input to similar information received in the past, creating some form of emotional response. If the emotional response is one of an alarming nature, then deeper-lying neurons are stimulated. This generally leads to a "fight or flight" reaction. For example, when someone who appears threatening approaches you and you feel endangered, you may freeze up or you may run away.

The emotion-laden information is also relayed to the frontal lobes, allowing the present experience to be integrated with experiences your brain has stored in memory.

This process forms the basis of the executive function of the frontal lobe, discussed in an earlier section. Properly functioning frontal lobes can integrate past and current experience, prevent "runaway emotional responses" and can logically organize and plan behavior that will enable you to work toward achieving the goals that you have set. The executive control system includes the ability to control the various aspects of attention.

Planning, logical and socially appropriate behavior, and a consciousness of the consequence of one's behavior are all functions largely controlled by these frontal lobes. If frontal lobe mechanisms fail, the result is impairment of attention and of impulse modulation and thinking itself.

When individuals with head injuries to the frontal lobes take psychological tests, they often display significant problems with the executive function of the frontal lobes. Yet their intellectual functioning or IQ scores remain surprisingly undisturbed. It is possible that some people with ADD were born with impaired frontal lobes (rather than incurring damage later).

Many researchers in the field of ADD suspect that the frontal lobes' inability to inhibit emotional responses and inappropriate behavior is what forms the very basis of this disease. The concept of "disinhibition of the frontal lobes" enjoys a fairly wide acceptance among researchers in this area.

Support for the frontal lobe theory comes from a wide variety of sources. Studies have revealed that individuals with attention deficit disorder typically have a widespread disorder of the frontal lobe function. They also share many features common to people who have suffered significant head trauma in which the frontal lobes were injured. When children with ADD are compared to children without ADD in *electroencephalograms* (brain wave studies), these studies reveal abnormal activity in the frontal lobes of the ADD children.

In his book *Anthropologists on Mars,* Oliver Sacks presents the history of Phineas Gage, an unfortunate gentleman who sustained a severe puncture wound extending into the frontal lobes. Miraculously, Mr. Gage survived the incident, although he was never quite "the same." The strange history was related by Mr. Gage's physician, John Martyn Harlow. Gage, Harlow writes, is

> . . . *fitful, irreverent, indulging at times in gross profanity (which was not previously his custom) manifesting little deference for his fellows, impatient with advice when it conflicts with his desires, at times pertinaciously obstinent, yet capricious and vacillating, devising many plans of future operations which are no longer ranged and then they are abandoned in term for others appearing more feasible. A child in his intellectual capacity and manifestations, he has the animal passions of a strong man. Previous to his injury, although untrained in the schools, he possessed a well balanced mind, and was looked upon by those who knew him as a shrewd, smart businessman, being energetic and persistent in executing all his plans of operation. In this regard, his mind was radically changed, so decidedly that his friends and acquaintances said he was "no longer Gage."*

One very exciting study on attention deficit disorder was reported by Zametkin, et al., in the prestigious *New England Journal of Medicine.* In this study, patients were examined using the exciting, advanced technology of the positron emission tomography (PET) scanning technique. PET scans, among other choices, can measure the use of glucose in the brain. Glucose is the primary source of energy for the brain, and following its consumption is constructive. As local activity in the brain increases, the amount of glucose used up also increases.

Adults with a history consistent with a diagnosis of attention deficit disorder and with at least one child diagnosed with attention deficit disorder were tested and compared to adults without ADD. This study showed beyond question that there was decreased consumption of glucose in precisely the hypothesized areas, i.e., the anterior portions of the frontal lobes. Other deeply lying areas of the brain also showed some diminished glucose metabolism.

It's also interesting to note that blood flow studies in people with attention deficit disorder have revealed a reduction of blood flow in precisely the frontal lobes. One study among many, reported in November 1995 by scientists at Emory University, reviewed PET scans on ten adult men, five diagnosed with ADD and five who did not have ADD. The men were given simple tasks to perform.

According to Dr. Julie Schweitzer, the blood flow differences were significant, as were the performance differences between the two groups. The blood flow in the information processing areas of the brain stayed high in the ADD men but fell off for the non-ADD men. In fact, Schweitzer stated that the ADD men worked harder. (Let's hope that everyone who has ever told an ADD person to "try harder" reads this.)

Schweitzer said the people with ADD need to first visualize the tasks they are given before they can perform, unlike people without ADD. Schweitzer also found that in patients treated with Ritalin, the blood flow was more normal and the patient performance on tests also improved.

MRI or CAT scans are tests that reveal the actual appearance of the brain rather than its function, and they have also demonstrated some very interesting abnormalities in the brains of boys with attention deficit disorder. Clear-cut anatomic abnormalities were observed in the frontal lobes, as well as in portions of the corpus callosum. (The corpus callosum is the bundle of nerve fibers connecting the two halves of the brain.) What researchers found with MRI studies was that the right frontal lobes were narrower in the individuals with ADD, compared to normal controls.

Other Areas of the Brain

Other researchers believe that other portions of the brain cause ADD—for example, the reticular activating system (RAS) and the locus coeruleus. These are deep-seated neuron systems. The reticular activating system is very important for the body's ability to remain alert. Impulses that reach the surface of the brain (the cortex), and keep them "primed," i.e., awake and receptive, actually originate in the reticular activating system. If this area is injured in animals, their alerting responses can be damaged and they also may become more distractible. This means they are not getting these important impulses to the cortex.

A group of neurons in the brainstem, called the locus coeruleus, appears to be the central component of the norepinephrine system. Norepinephrine is another neurotransmitter in the catecholamine series. Some researchers believe that in people with ADD, the locus coeruleus is "firing" at an increased rate. Some medications that are suspected of reducing the firing rate of the locus coeruleus have also been effective in the treatment of attention deficit disorder, including the tricyclic antidepressants and clonidine.

The Theory of Dopamine Deficiency Syndrome

A fascinating article by Bloom et al., published in *American Scientist,* presented evidence linking a dopamine receptor (D2) deficiency state to a broad spectrum of behavioral abnormalities including alcoholism, attention deficit disorder, drug abuse and/or food bingeing, and pathologic gambling. The authors hypothesized that an abnormality in the dopamine system leads to an impaired ability to achieve a sense of well-being, which the authors called "the ultimate reward."

The authors discuss the work of James Old, an American psychologist who mistakenly placed an electrode in limbic system structures deep in the brain of some rats. When the rats were able to activate this electrode themselves, they would press the lever up to 5,000 times an hour and would only interrupt this autostimulation to sleep. The animals would endure hardship and severe and prolonged pain in order to pursue this pleasurable stimulation.

These researchers believe that dopamine is the primary neurotransmitter involving this type of reward behavior. They describe various experiments performed on selectively bred strains of rats that preferred drinking alcohol to water. These "party animals" had a low number of dopamine D2 receptors in their limbic systems. Drugs that stimulated the D2 receptor caused the rats to cut back on their alcohol ingestion. Conversely, drugs that blocked this receptor would make them go "off the wagon."

The study also presented data on the abnormal D2 gene in humans. In comparing severe alcoholics to nonalcoholics, the researchers found the abnormal gene in 69 percent of the alcoholics. It was present in only 20 percent of nonalcoholics.

In looking at human cocaine addicts, the abnormal D2 receptor gene was present in 52 percent of cocaine addicts and only 21 percent of nonaddicts. In people with attention deficit disorder, the abnormal D2 receptor gene was present in 49 percent of the children studied with attention deficit disorder, compared to only 27 percent of the children who did not have ADD.

In one study reported in 1995 in the *American Journal of Human Genetics,* researchers found a linkage between attention deficit disorder and the dopamine transporter gene. We believe that the abnormal D2 receptor gene contributes to such disorders as alcoholism, addiction, and ADD, but other genetic abnormalities, as well as environmental factors, also have significant influence on the individual.

Other studies suggest that yet another dopamine receptor (D4 receptor) might be related to another form of ADD-like behavior, "novelty seeking." Overactivity leads to obsessive-compulsive disorder while underactivity leads to ADD.

Scientists have also found a specific gene in some children with attention deficit disorder, it was announced in April 1996. They found the gene in 49 percent of children with attention deficit hyperactivity disorder but in only 21 percent of children without ADHD. They also found the children with the genetic variant showed more ADD-like symptoms than did the children with attention deficit disorder but without the gene.

An April 1996 announcement by Dr. Paul Manowitz, Associate Professor of Psychiatry and Neurology at the University of Medicine and Dentistry of New Jersey, reported yet another genetic defect in alcoholics. Dr. Manowitz has suggested that a deficiency in an enzyme called arylsulfatase A might be related to alcoholism, as well as behavior problems such as attention deficits, impulsivity, hyperactivity, emotional instability, and poor judgment. An enzyme is a helper protein that allows a chemical process to occur in a rapid orderly fashion. Enzyme deficiencies can cause many diseases, including some types of mental retardation.

The Theory of ADD As a Social Invention

We do not believe that ADD is caused by society or by bad parenting, as some claim, with scant evidence. For example, a perplexing article authored by Thomas Armstrong, Ph.D., appeared in *Education Week* in October 1995. In this strange treatise, Armstrong takes to task those who readily accept what he sees as the mythical fantasy of ADD. He also chastises people for not being able to see the "bigger picture."

According to Armstrong, attention deficit disorder is part conspiracy and part an expression of a very sick society. He perceives attention deficit disorder as a paralytic attempt by an unjust society to legitimize itself. Armstrong also compares ADD to a mythical disease described in 1851 by a Louisiana physician, Dr. Samuel A. Cartwright. Dr. Cartwright had proposed a medical theory to explain runaway slaves which he called "drapetomania." Armstrong says modern society labels its "attention runaways" as suffering from a medical condition in the tradition of the erstwhile slave owners.

Leaving common sense far behind, Armstrong offensively compares individuals suffering from this neurologic disorder to the sentinel canaries that were placed in mine shafts to alert miners of an inadequate oxygen supply in the mine. (If there wasn't enough oxygen, the canaries would die, thereby alerting miners to evacuate.)

Armstrong's thesis about ADD also contained an irrelevant racial slant. This ingenious "invention," according to Armstrong, is the ultimate weapon of America's bigoted class society and will allow ADD special education to be the battering ram to de-mainstream minorities seeking to access our country's educational resources. Armstrong closes with the heartfelt lament that these "issues" raised in his article are not commonly discussed in the debate surrounding attention deficit disorder.

We take great issue with the concept of attention deficit disorder as an attempt by society to disempower a large portion of the population and to target this group for wanton exploitation. We regard Dr. Armstrong as being the Lawrence Welk of the aging counterculture, mystified by what he sees and denying the existence of what should be perfectly obvious, while belting out the philosophical golden oldies about a cruel and greedy society that places self-justification above children and privilege above the nation's future.

Genetics-Based Studies and Theories

Genetic studies of individuals and families have provided some interesting data on attention deficit disorder. These studies have provided very cogent arguments that this syndrome is, at least in part, hereditary.

Adoption studies provide information on the relative importance of upbringing (nurture) vs. genetic factors (nature). These studies typically involved detailed psychiatric analysis of an adoptee's biological as well as adoptive families. These studies have indicated that the development of attention deficit disorder is very highly correlated with the biological parents and has very little to do with the family that actually reared the child.

These studies have also dealt a very powerful blow to those who insist that attention deficit disorder is a purely behavioral disturbance and is a consequence of "bad parenting."

Genetic studies have also uncovered the remarkable fact that relatives of individuals with attention deficit disorder have a much higher incidence of anxiety and depressive illnesses than do individuals without this disorder. In addition, studies on identical twins have indicated that there is a much higher risk for ADD in identical twins than in nonidentical twin pairs. Identical twins carry essentially the same genetic material while nonidentical twins do not.

Possible Environmental Causes

We believe that the actual syndrome of attention deficit disorder is a complex interplay of environmental and genetic factors. But what environmental factors appear to be relevant?

Generally, this type of discussion starts with von Economo's encephalitis, a virus that raged throughout the world in the 1920s, affecting both children and adults. After they recovered from this disease, many adults developed a syndrome that was clinically indistinguishable from Parkinson's disease, while the children developed syndromes consistent with a diagnosis of attention deficit disorder and conduct disorders.

This finding has led to a search for other environmentally related injuries, particularly to the young brain, and which result in the later appearance of this syndrome. Various complications of birth, low birth weight, cigarette-smoking mothers, seizures during pregnancy, prematurity, as well as head trauma and viral encephalitis, have all been correlated with attention deficit disorder. However, no specific mechanism or causal agent has yet been identified.

There are still those people who blame bad parents or a bad school or home life for attention deficit disorder. There is very little support for this view. It is true that ineffective parents can cause children to be unhappy; however, rarely can they cause hyperactivity, distractibility, and other symptoms seen in ADD. It's also possible that the parents themselves have ADD, and if the child has ADD too, the disorder was transmitted genetically.

Other Theories of Causes

Some researchers have found a linkage between a rare form of thyroid disease and attention deficit disorder. A study on this topic was reported in a 1993 issue of *The New England Journal of Medicine*. The disorder causes the person to have a resistance to thyroid hormone and can result in hyperactivity and other ADD symptoms.

In their study of children and adults with this thyroid hormone resistance, half of the adults with this thyroid problem also had ADD. According to the study, only 7 percent of the adults with normal thyroid responses had ADD. A huge 70 percent of the children with the thyroid problem had ADD, versus only 20 percent of the children with normal thyroid reactions.

Some scientists have found children with underactive thyroid glands to behave in a hyperactive manner. Presumably, the brain causes an overstimulation to compensate for the understimulation of the thyroid gland. This is probably not a common contributing factor in ADD. While thyroid disease is common, the direct causal relationship between thyroid disease and ADD has not been clearly established at this time.

We feel many factors can combine to cause the development of ADD and ADD is probably a nonspecific biochemical and developmental response to a wide variety of disease-causing processes.

3

Diagnosing ADD

"Sometimes a cigar is just a cigar."   —Sigmund Freud

"Anyone who goes to a psychiatrist ought to have his
head examined."   —Samuel Goldwyn

The cornerstone for the effective treatment of any disease
is a proper diagnosis. Beginning treatment before completing an accurate diagnosis can be very dangerous for the
patient. Yet for someone with ADD, the necessary logical and
methodical approach might seem about as tedious as reading
the phone book. You need to be patient and understand that
many illnesses could be confused with ADD, and it's very
unwise to rush to judgment with a diagnosis.

To illustrate, let's look at another common illness, diabetes. Undiagnosed patients with diabetes frequently com-
plain of fatigue and an excessive need to urinate and to drink
fluids. While these symptoms are quite suggestive of diabetes, what patient would be satisfied if the physician ran no

tests and did no careful analysis, but instead immediately presented the patient with hypodermic needles, insulin, a home glucose testing apparatus—and a bill? If the patient did *not* have diabetes but were treated as if she did, she would be more than inconvenienced. Administering insulin unnecessarily could be fatal.

This analogy is somewhat extreme, but it's true that serious consequences could occur to a patient hurriedly diagnosed as having ADD when the actual cause might actually be another undiagnosed medical condition.

The Diagnostic Process

The diagnostic process for ADD, as well as for any other medical condition, must begin with a formal medical history. The physician will ask the patient, and possibly family members, about early developmental history, trauma, and a whole host of various symptoms and medical conditions. A general physical examination should be conducted in which blood pressure is checked, heart and lungs are examined, etc. The physical examination may indicate a need for further testing, such as X rays and blood tests. In order to exclude the many neurologic conditions that can mimic the ADD symptom complex, a formal neurologic assessment by a neurologist should also be a part of this physical examination.

Remember that the diagnostic process is a "joint venture" between the patient and the physician, requiring patience, honesty, and commitment from both parties.

Diagnosis of Attention Deficit Disorder in Adults

The diagnosis of attention deficit disorder in adults is a very complex undertaking. It is based on some positive criteria such as hyperactivity and impulsivity, but also on negative criteria. "Negative criteria" refers to the absence of any alternative medical condition that could manifest in similar ways. If no other medical explanation for the patient's behavior can be identified, then the diagnosis will be based primarily on the presence of symptoms reported by the patient and/or other individuals who might know the patient, i.e. family, friends, etc., and performance on various neuropsychological testing.

The American Psychiatric Association periodically publishes an updated manual of diagnostic criteria for various mental conditions in which behavioral abnormalities are prominent. The most recent edition of this manual as of this writing is the *Diagnostic and Statistical Manual IV (DSM-IV)*, and it includes guidelines for the diagnosis of attention deficit disorder. We have enclosed the portion of this manual relevant to attention deficit disorder for the reader's examination. *It should be noted that* DSM-IV *is for experienced professionals and is not intended for self-diagnosis of attention deficit disorder or any other condition treated in the manual.*

A. Either (1) or (2):
    (1) Inattention: at least 6 of the following symptoms of inattention have persisted for at least 6 months to a degree that is maladaptive and inconsistent with developmental level:
    (a) often fails to give close attention to details or makes careless mistakes in schoolwork, work, or other activities
    (b) often has difficulty sustaining attention in tasks or play activities
    (c) often does not seem to listen to what is being said to him/her
    (d) often does not follow through on instructions and fails to finish schoolwork, chores, or duties in the workplace (not due to oppositional behavior or failure to understand instructions)

(e) often has difficulties organizing tasks and activities

(f) often avoids or strongly dislikes tasks (such as schoolwork or homework) that require sustained mental effort

(g) often loses things necessary for tasks or activities (e.g., school assignments, pencils, books, tools, or toys)

(h) is often easily distracted by extraneous stimuli

(i) often forgetful in daily activities

(2) Hyperactivity-impulsivity: at least 4 of the following symptoms of hyperactivity-impulsivity have persisted for at least 6 months to a degree that is maladaptive and inconsistent with developmental level:

Hyperactivity:

(a) often fidgets with hands or feet or squirms in seat

(b) leaves seat in classroom or in other situations in which remaining seated is expected

(c) often runs about or climbs excessively in situations where it is inappropriate (in adolescents or adults, may be limited to subjective feelings of restlessness)

(d) often has difficulty playing or engaging in leisure activities quietly

Impulsivity:

(e) often blurts out answers to questions before the questions have been completed

(f) often has difficulty waiting in lines or awaiting turn in games or group situations

B. Onset no later than age 7.

C. Symptoms must be present in 2 or more situations (e.g., at school, work, and at home).

D. The disturbance causes clinically significant distress or impairment in social, academic, or occu-
pational functioning.
E. Does not occur exclusively during the course of
PDD, schizophrenia or other psychotic disorder,
and is not better accounted for by mood, anxiety,
dissociative, or personality disorder.

Based on the information in this reference, individuals are
coded as "ADHD, Predominantly Inattentive Type if criterion
A(1) is met but not criterion A(2) for the past 6 months," or they
are "ADHD, Predominantly Hyperactive-Impulsive Type: if criterion A(2) is met but not criterion A(1) for the past 6 months."

In addition, a third category, "ADHD Combined Type," is
diagnosed if "both criteria A(1) and (2) are met for past 6
months."[1]

There are certain shortcomings in the *DSM-IV.* These
guidelines often fall short of the mark in specific areas, usually
in the form of underdiagnosis. As a result, further testing in
the form of neuropsychological evaluation can be very useful.

The diagnostic dilemma of adult attention deficit disorder
is primarily related to the great difficulty of obtaining a history of relevant ADD childhood behaviors, because part of
diagnosis is determining whether the onset of symptoms
occurred before the patient was age seven.

A forty-year-old—or even a twenty-five-year-old—may
have a difficult time remembering back to childhood. If a
family member, such as a parent, is available for questioning,
then documenting childhood symptoms is typically easier.
However, some family members are hesitant and defensive
to describe some of the behaviors they observed in the
patient because of embarrassment, unwillingness to accept
the diagnosis, and possible sensations of guilt. There might
be one more factor: the informant may have ADD as well.

---

1. The above information was quoted here with the written permission of the
American Psychiatric Association.

Persons suffering from attention deficit disorder can be very difficult for a doctor to work with in that they are frequently late, disorganized, and occasionally antisocial. Add to this that the patient may have other behavioral or psychiatric problems (called "co-morbidity") that might be much more severe than attention deficit disorder and may include depression, substance abuse, or other symptoms. Or he may have been diagnosed with another problem when his true underlying problem is ADD.

The following illustrates this problem.

Alex B., a 28-year-old man, was referred to our neurologic clinic for evaluation after he reported to the local emergency room for a second time, having had a generalized convulsion. The patient had already had an MRI scan of the brain, as well as an electroencephalogram. Both were normal. Alex was accompanied by his mother, who was quite concerned about her son's condition. Alex spoke somewhat unclearly, as he had bitten the tip of his tongue severely during the seizure.

Careful questioning of the patient and his mother revealed that Alex had a serious drinking problem and that the two episodes of seizures had occurred shortly after terminations of these drinking episodes. Interestingly, Alex had been seen by another neurologist locally who had specifically asked about alcohol abuse, which Alex had denied.

During our interview, we noticed that Alex was very anxious, disorganized, and fidgeting. Moreover, he was thirty minutes late for his appointment, despite his mother having arrived punctually. Further questioning suggested that Alex actually had attention deficit disorder. He was subsequently tested, found to have the disorder, and was ultimately treated with Ritalin.

Dramatically, Alex no longer has a drinking problem, nor has he had any further seizures. The proper diagnosis and treatment resolved his problems. The frightening part about all this is that a physician

*uninformed about ADD often would diagnose Alex with
epilepsy, in the absence of the history of alcoholism and
attention deficit disorder. [Remember that Alex had lied
about his drinking problem.] If he had been diagnosed
with epilepsy, then Alex would normally be put on an
anticonvulsant drug. The probability is very high that
such treatment would have made his ADD symptoms
much worse.*

(For more on similarities between ADD and epilepsy, see chapter 4.)

Bad Parenting Does Not Cause ADD, but ADD Can Contribute to Bad Parenting

A remarkable presentation of adult attention deficit disorder was presented by Daly and Fritsch. An infant was hospitalized twice during his second month of life because of poor feeding. The usual diagnostic studies were performed, but demonstrated no evidence of organic disease. After the second hospitalization, a pediatric psychiatry team got involved. The team quickly identified the mother as having severe attention deficit disorder. Successful treatment of the mother with methylphenidate (Ritalin) enabled the mother to give closer attention to her baby.

Neuropsychological Testing

Neuropsychological tests are employed in research and in the evaluation of individuals suspected of having attention deficit disorder. In addition, there are multiple screening questionnaires used by clinicians. Screening questionnaires can be valuable for the diagnosis of ADD and can also suggest the presence of other behavioral disturbances, such as depression and anxiety.

The Wender Utah Rating Scale is often used in the diagnostic evaluation of individuals suspected of having attention deficit disorder. This is a questionnaire study focusing on childhood behavior and provides little information about the adult's current functioning, for instance in relationships and at work.

An adult ADHD questionnaire developed by Nadeau includes nineteen specific categories which are assessed, including inattention, hyperactivity, anger control, and academic performance. In each category, fifteen or fewer questions are administered while the patient rates the applicability on a scale of 0–4.

IQ testing is often used as a tool in diagnosing attention deficit disorder. While it is generally agreed among researchers and clinicians that the diagnosis of attention deficit disorder is not directly related to intelligence, the finding of normal intelligence would exclude various other medical conditions that could superficially be confused with attention deficit disorder.[2]

The Wechsler Adult Intelligence Scale, revised (WAIS-R), is commonly used for this purpose. The Test of Variables of Attention computer program (T.O.V.A.) is one of the continuous process tests in which attention can be assessed. The subject is presented with a repetitive task and instructed to watch for targets and ignore nontargets. The Conners Test is a similar test for attention.

The T.O.V.A. and Conners tests both assess attention based on visual input, while another continuous process test, the Comprehensive Auditory Visual Attention Assessment System, assesses visual and auditory attention. Many other tests exist in which attention, impulsivity, memory, and ability to plan and execute tasks are assessed, but the discussion of these individual tests would be beyond the scope of this book.

---

2. One caveat to this approach is that an individual with ADD can often score deceptively low on IQ testing for various reasons, including difficulty concentrating, anxiety, or failure to understand instructions.

How Do People Feel When They Are Diagnosed?

Many people are diagnosed after they notice they are exhibiting the same symptoms as their children who are diagnosed with ADD. So they are not surprised to learn they have ADD. Others first learn about ADD when they see a program on TV or read an article in a newspaper or magazine. Sometimes other people tell them about ADD.

The reactions of people who are diagnosed with ADD vary, but many say they feel relief that the problem finally has a name. Said one person, "Before diagnosis and treatment, I felt the constant blackness of dissatisfaction and the restlessness of feeling unfulfilled. When I was diagnosed at the age of thirty-four, I was relieved but I also had to overcome being sad over the lost years. Now I'm learning to cope."

Said another person, "I was relieved that I was a normal human being and that it could be effectively treated." And, from a woman with ADD who was diagnosed at the age of thirty-five, "I knew there was something wrong but I couldn't figure out what. This gave me a logical explanation as to why I couldn't seem to do certain things, why I couldn't seem to finish anything I started. ADD was explained to me in a way that didn't make me feel 'inferior' to the rest of humanity."

Often people have mixed feelings about being diagnosed with ADD, perhaps relief mixed with sadness. Said Susan K., "It's hard to walk the line between feeling flawed and feeling like I'm just wired differently."

4

Differential Diagnosis and "Co-Morbidities"

When Something Else Looks Like (or Another Problem Accompanies) ADD

———⟨⟨⟨⟨⟨ § ⟩⟩⟩⟩⟩———

To know what attention deficit disorder is, you also need to know what it is *not,* and a good physician considers other possible psychiatric and neurologic problems that a person with distractibility, inattention, and other ADD symptoms may have. Other factors should be considered, too, such as the person's age and already existing medical problems.

For example, when an otherwise healthy young adult goes to see a doctor and complains of a cough, diagnosis is usually easy. The physician will ask basic questions and perform a physical examination. Sometimes X rays and laboratory studies will be ordered too. The diagnosis will often be acute bronchitis, which responds very well to medical treatment.

But if that same person comes in many years later complaining about a new cough, diagnosis may be more difficult. At that point she may have other illnesses alongside the primary diagnosis. (The presence of such secondary or accompanying problems is called *co-morbidity.*) In the case of the person with the persistent cough, the cough *could* be caused by bronchitis, but the patient may also have other illnesses as well that are contributing to and complicating the problem.

The *differential diagnosis* is a list of various conditions that a physician needs to consider before making a final diagnosis. In the case of an older, frail individual with a severe cough, the differential diagnosis could include many conditions that need to be ruled out by the doctor, such as acute bronchitis, malignancy, congestive heart failure, and potential side effects of a medication.

Similarly, when an adult comes to a physician with symptoms of ADD, it's also very important to look at other possible causes for the inattention, hyperactivity, distractibility, and other symptoms that may mimic attention deficit disorder. It's also true that the older the individual being considered for the diagnosis of ADD, the more likely it is that some other condition (such as depression) may coexist in this same individual. By the same token, the older a person gets, the more likely it is that *other* conditions may be responsible for the ADD-like symptoms that have led her to seek the doctor's help.

In this chapter, we discuss illnesses that may be confused by psychologists or other physicians with ADD, including post-traumatic stress disorder, AIDS, and Lyme disease. To further complicate the diagnostic challenge, many people with ADD have "co-morbid" (coexisting) problems on top of the ADD. As a result, we are including information on many illnesses that often accompany ADD, such as depression and anxiety.

Post-Traumatic Stress Disorder

Post-traumatic stress disorder (PTSD—also called *post-traumatic stress syndrome*) occurs frequently after combat, rape, assault, or some other severe traumatic experience, and affects about 3 percent of the population. Obviously, some type of predisposition must be present in the patient, because many people experience extreme psychological trauma without developing such a cataclysmic response. It is important to note that the severity of the inciting event does not always correlate with the degree of reaction. People react differently to traumatic events, and one person might react severely while another adjusts relatively quickly.

What can cause post-traumatic stress syndrome? Childhood mistreatment, a preexisting psychologic disturbance such as personality disorder, alcohol abuse, and other factors appear to predispose individuals to developing this disorder when faced with a traumatic event such as a wartime experience or personal assault. Post-traumatic stress disorder causes the person to actively avoid experiences that might remind him of the stressful episode. But even avoiding such experiences won't resolve the problem, and the person often will have intrusive thoughts related to the stressful event. The individual with post-traumatic stress syndrome is often described as being hypervigilant, unable to relax, and always on guard. A delay of several years can occur between the traumatic event and the symptoms of this disorder.

What does PTSD have to do with attention deficit disorder? Many of their symptoms overlap. For example, a person with each problem may experience an impaired sense of their surroundings, a feeling of being "different." Each may exhibit avoidance behavior, anxiety, and work and academic underachievement. Difficulty concentrating is another symptom shared by people with each disorder.

What is different is that generally in the case of a person with PTSD, there's no history of impulsivity, hyperactivity, inattention, and distractibility. Also, the extreme emotional event leading to this disorder can usually be identified. Yet sometimes this event may seem fairly trivial in nature and may be difficult to identify. As a result, distinguishing between attention deficit disorder and post-traumatic stress syndrome can be a very difficult undertaking.

Neurologic Illnesses with ADD-Like Symptoms

We discussed the frontal lobes in chapter 2 and cited the example of Phineas Gage. The frontal lobes can be affected by a variety of medical conditions and injuries, of which head injury is the most common.

The frontal lobes are particularly prone to injury and head trauma, as are the temporal lobes. Because of their vulnerable locations, even a slight displacement can injure brain tissue. Aside from trauma, the frontal lobes can also be affected by tumors, strokes, infections, degenerative diseases, as well as by disturbance of the normal flow of the cerebrospinal fluid (the fluid surrounding the brain).

Chronic alcohol abuse can severely affect the frontal lobes, and conditions such as multiple sclerosis may also lead to problems in frontal lobe function. Dysfunction of the frontal lobes may also be involved in depression, obsessive/compulsive disorders, and even schizophrenia. In the not so recent past, the frontal lobes were selectively damaged by neurosurgeons (frontal lobotomy) in an effort to "custodialize" difficult psychiatric patients.

Frontal Lobe Disease

Anton S. was a twenty-five-year-old man who sought our services because of a dramatic change in his behavior. He was essentially "dragged" to see a neurologist because of alteration in his judgment, social inappropriateness of behavior, and memory impairment. He also complained of some very mild headaches, particularly in the early morning hours.

On neurological examination, we found Anton had some memory difficulties, as well as difficulties completing tasks. We saw other evidence of frontal lobe dysfunction of both lobes. Anton underwent a CT scan, which raised some suspicion about an abnormality near the base of the brain. Because of the overwhelming suspicion of bifrontal lobe disease, we ordered an MRI, which revealed a large benign tumor at the base of the frontal lobes.

Anton had surgery and most of his symptoms abated. What does this have to do with ADD? Individuals suffering from frontal lobe disease also have problems with attention, social appropriateness, judgment/insight, emotional responses, and the ability to complete tasks.

The disease can be identified using various tests, including electroencephalograms and imaging studies. The patient's mental history is also of great importance.

Epilepsy

Epilepsy—a seizure disorder—is another disease that a doctor should rule out before diagnosing ADD. There are many types of epilepsies, but the two most relevant and likely to be confused with ADD are *petit mal* epilepsy seizures and *complex partial* seizures.

In petit mal seizures, the patient temporarily loses consciousness while maintaining body tone. Some fumbling with the fingers is occasionally seen. During the actual spells, the patient has no ability to form new memories or to interact with anyone.

Very commonly, this form of epilepsy is identified in childhood and treated appropriately. Patients often stop having spells by adulthood, but many go on to have different types of seizures. Electroencephalography is particularly helpful in identifying this type of seizure.

Untreated individuals with this type of disorder will have many of the problems commonly encountered in attention deficit disorder, including memory impairment and underachievement in academic and professional settings.

The complex partial seizure is another form of epilepsy and is similar to petit mal seizures. Frequently, the patient will stare off into space for a few seconds or a few minutes, and appear to be out of touch with her surroundings. An adult with ADD who is hyperfocusing might look like a person with this disorder. Occasionally, this seizure will develop into a generalized convulsive episode, which is not hard to diagnose.

These events occur primarily due to injury to the temporal lobes, but can only occur after injury to other lobes such as the frontal. The patient will usually have no recollection of having a seizure. There may be some confusion lasting for several minutes after a spell of this type.

During the seizure the patient may be able to chew gum or even hold objects in the hand and will frequently continue acts that were begun prior to the seizure. As with petit mal seizures, this type of episodic lapse in consciousness can lead to serious functional and social impairment. The nineteenth-century Russian novelist Fyodor Dostoyevsky was thought to suffer from this form of epilepsy.

A patient can become quite violent during a seizure. His violence is usually, however, related to attempts by observers to subdue him.

While most individuals with complex partial seizures are normal between the attacks, many of them will have behavioral problems outside the actual seizure episodes. Individuals may have obsessive tendencies, particularly in the sphere of religious activities, sexual disturbances, and even psychosis.

The diagnosis of complex partial seizures is simply made on the basis of atypical EEG findings, as well as other abnormalities on neurological examination and a history of a "spell" suggestive of a seizure. The ADD features of impulsivity and hyperactivity are usually absent. Naturally, attention is seriously compromised during the spells themselves. Typically, there is no childhood history of symptoms characteristic of attention deficit disorder.

Acquired Immune Deficiency Syndrome (AIDS)

The *acquired immune deficiency syndrome* (AIDS) is a constellation of various types of manifestations of an impaired immune system, leading to an increased susceptibility to and frequency of infections and malignancies. AIDS is a consequence of infections with the *human immunodeficiency virus*

(HIV). This virus is usually contracted through sexual inter-course with an infected person, and individuals who have many sexual partners are at much greater risk for contracting HIV than are those who are actively involved with one part-ner (who is faithful to them) or those who are celibate.

Over half the patients suffering from AIDS will have sig-nificant neurologic disease by the time of their death. Evi-dence of brain dysfunction will be the main symptom of AIDS in less than 5 percent of the cases. However, perhaps 50 per-cent of patients acquiring this disorder will have dementia by the time of death.

While HIV virus leads to susceptibility to various other infections and even malignancies, and these are usually the illnesses that seriously sicken or kill the person, the HIV virus itself is responsible for most of the neurologic disease in the brain.

Patients with a spread of the disease to the brain com-plain of compromised intellectual function, fatigue, head-aches, the loss of sex drive, and many will have seizures. The parallel to ADD is that forgetfulness, difficulty concen-trating, and difficulty completing tasks are all symptoms shared by both people with ADD and those afflicted with HIV infection.

So how do you tell them apart? Usually, the distinction is based on history. The ADDer will have the usual childhood manifestations of the disease, while the AIDS patient will not. However, as we noted above, the HIV sufferer may have fairly profound disturbance in memory, which could make obtain-ing a reliable history very difficult.

Other clear-cut symptoms exist. Often at the time of diagnosis, the HIV-infected individual will have muscle wast-ing, loss of hair, and enlarged glands, and imaging studies will reveal a shrunken brain. Of course, the HIV blood test will be positive in the person with the virus. The person with ADD will not show such symptoms, unless the person has ADD *and* HIV.

Tourette's Syndrome

Tourette's syndrome affects over 100,000 Americans. It has considerable overlap with attention deficit disorder and is probably the neurologic disease with the highest degree of co-morbidity with ADD. Approximately half of the patients with Tourette's also fulfill the diagnostic criteria of attention deficit disorder. (Almost as many with Tourette's syndrome are also found to have obsessive/compulsive disorder.)

Both motor and vocal tics are usually found with this illness (involuntary motor or vocal outbursts). The motor tics often consist of blinking, grimacing, jerking motions of the extremities, clearing the throat, and sighing. These tics generally appear at the age of seven. The vocal tics may appear somewhat later. The vocal tics cause the person to involuntarily speak profane or insulting words to people, leading to virtual social isolation in many cases. Difficulties with attention, impulsivity, and other ADD-type symptoms frequently complicate the disorder.

As with attention deficit disorder, this childhood-onset condition appears to be hereditary and it continues into adulthood. Unlike attention deficit disorder, the symptoms of Tourette's syndrome frequently wax and wane in severity.

Other Problems That May Mimic ADD

Beyond the quite numerous illnesses that traditionally have fallen into the realm of psychiatry and neurology, a number of other states and conditions deserve mention. One of these would be drug toxicity. A number of medications, such as antihistamines, various cardiac medications, and sedatives can lead to poor concentration, impaired judgment, and attention-related problems. Drug use, particularly cocaine abuse, is another such problem, as are various endocrine disorders such as hypoglycemia and thyroid disease. The formal and exhaustive medical evaluation can prevent an individual from being erroneously labeled as an ADDer and thus be wrongly treated with medications and other interventions. Recognition of the mimicking illness can thereby be recognized and subsequently treated appropriately.

Lyme Disease

In the not-so-distant past, many people who suffered from the bite of the Lyme tick went undiagnosed, and doctors thought they were basically faking their symptoms. Now we have a test for Lyme disease, but, of course, it must be administered by a physician.

What does this have to do with ADD? According to an October 1995 issue of the *Harvard Mental Health Letter,* among other symptoms, cognitive deficits occur with Lyme disease, such as the "loss of the ability to sustain attention on tasks." Studies have also revealed that children afflicted with Lyme disease may also experience hyperactivity and have trouble concentrating.

If a person afflicted with Lyme disease were misdiagnosed with ADD, as could happen, then that person would be treated improperly, and all the counseling and Ritalin in the world wouldn't help much—and could be harmful. As a result, Lyme disease is one ailment that should be ruled out by your doctor. This is another reason why you should be diagnosed by a *medical doctor* rather than by a psychologist or therapist, who probably would not recognize the symptoms of Lyme disease and would not be able to order the necessary tests even if she did.

Thyroid Disease

In chapter 2, on causes of ADD, we discussed several possible links to thyroid disease; however, it is also possible that a person could have a thyroid disease and not have ADD. For this reason, any person who seems unusually hyperactive and inattentive should probably be evaluated by a physician for possible thyroid disease.

Alzheimer's Disease

Although most people think of Alzheimer's disease as a medical problem faced by people over age sixty-five, it is possible for a person in middle age to have this disease. Because the illness is characterized by forgetfulness and confusion, and because the early onset may be mild, it is possible that this problem could be misdiagnosed as the inattentive form of ADD.

It is a good idea to see a neurologist who can rule out this illness as well as the others discussed in this chapter, because there are medications that can help people with Alzheimer's; it is no longer considered an untreatable problem.

When Other Illnesses Coexist with ADD

It is also possible, as mentioned at the beginning of this chapter, that you could have attention deficit disorder *and* another medical problem, and this section of the chapter discusses such possible "co-morbid" disorders.

In one study of adults with ADD, reported in *A Comprehensive Guide to Attention Deficit Disorder in Adults,* the authors reported on 114 adults attending an ADD clinic. Forty-one percent of the adults had one or more disorders in addition to the ADD. Interestingly, 61 percent had some significant co-morbid condition at some other point in their lives, and 38 percent of the individuals were found to have two or more co-morbid conditions.

(*Note:* This does not mean that you must have another problem in addition to ADD. Your ADD may very well be the sole problem you are experiencing. Others, however, have also had other serious problems. The figures above simply indicate the frequency of co-morbidity.)

In an article in the December 1995 issue of the *American Journal of Psychiatry*, the specific additional illnesses studied were major depression, bipolar disorder, and generalized anxiety disorder. The authors were able to eliminate the various symptoms that ADD shares with the other co-morbidities and examine the remaining symptoms for adequate features of the various conditions to fulfill the precise diagnostic criteria for the various co-morbid states. The authors concluded that after removing the shared symptoms/features, 79 percent of patients had a valid diagnosis of major depression, bipolar disorder, or generalized anxiety disorder based on the data remaining. These studies indicate very clearly that these conditions are actually coexisting with attention deficit disorder.

We will discuss psychiatric conditions that may exist concurrently in one person. We would like to emphasize that the co-morbidities may be far worse than the attention deficit disorder, and a combination of these co-morbidities can be infinitely more debilitating than any of the single diagnoses by themselves and can lead to considerable health risks, including abuse of psychoactive substances.

Depression

Depression is a very common disorder in western society, and contains many features that will overlap with the symptoms of attention deficit disorder. Many individuals think suicide is the most extreme expression of depression; however, depression can become so severe that the individual is in a stupor, and is unmotivated to eat, speak, or attend to bodily functions. In extreme depression, the patient is too debilitated to commit suicide.

In addition to an overall depressed mood, there are other diagnostic criteria for depression.

- Lack of motivation
- Changes in social interaction
- Loss of interest in hobbies

* Change in eating or sleeping patterns
* Lack of energy
* Low self-esteem
* Preoccupation with death

The disordered sleep pattern that is seen in depression frequently involves early morning awakening with an inability to fall asleep again, or sleeping in excess.

Persons with ADD tend to have rapidly changing thoughts and ideas, which interferes with falling asleep or maintaining sleep. It is here that the uncovering of a lifelong pattern of underachievement, procrastination, failure to complete tasks, and other symptoms of ADD is very important in differentiating from the more episodic nature of the depressive state.

Dysthymia is another depressive illness in which the symptoms of depression are present more than two years. In one study reported by Shekim and others, ten percent of the adults in an ADD clinic also carried the diagnosis of major depression, while 25 percent were diagnosed as suffering from dysthymia.

In some people, the co-morbid condition of depression may be a consequence of attention deficit disorder and may become much more troubling to the patient than the underlying problem, i.e. ADD.

Bipolar Disorder

Bipolar disorder, also known as *manic depression,* is also seen in people with ADD. A person without ADD who has bipolar disorder may appear as though she has ADD. This is why a careful diagnosis is very important.

Bipolar disorder is a condition in which episodes of mania and depression alternate. The manic phase shows many of the symptoms of attention deficit disorder, such as impaired attention, distractibility, restlessness, mood variation, "flightiness," and rapid and often pressured speech. What is different about bipolar disorder is the cyclical nature of the illness. The symptoms of attention deficit disorder are usually much more pervasive and longer-lasting.

The manic phase in bipolar disorder can last for months, while the mood swings and irascibility in attention deficit disorder tend to be much more short-lived, i.e., hours to days. A family history of bipolar disorder is more common in close relatives of bipolar-disordered individuals than in the relatives of people with attention deficit disorder. (And there is also a strong probability that people with ADD have close relatives with ADD. It's just that the probability is higher with bipolar disorder.)

Anxiety Disorders

Anxiety disorders are frequently seen in individuals with attention deficit disorder, and they often confuse the diagnosis. A person who does not have ADD, but is a relative of a person with ADD, is at risk for suffering from an anxiety disorder.

The *DSM-IV* recognizes ten different types of anxiety disorders, but we will discuss only the ones more relative to our current discussion. The disorders we'll discuss have an enormous degree of overlap with ADD.

Individuals suffering from generalized anxiety disorder, while free of actual panic attacks, tend to have anxiety as a dominant feature of their emotional lives. These individuals fret and worry about any number of concerns of their daily life.

Individuals with ADD are often fairly accomplished worriers, and this may be one of the most debilitating features of the illness. Women are twice as prone to suffer from anxiety as are men. Unfortunately, only about one-third of the patients suffering from this disorder eventually seek psychiatric treatment. Patients with generalized anxiety disorder are frequently seen in the offices of general practitioners, cardiologists, gastroenterologists . . . and neurologists. Individuals

with generalized anxiety disorder may be restless, hypervigilant, and demonstrate rapid heartbeat and inordinate sweating. Startling one of these individuals can send him "through
the roof." They will typically lack the impulsivity, disorganization, and attention failure seen in ADD. Phobias represent
another subcategory of anxiety disorders, but typically are
very easily differentiated from ADD, as the phobia is typically
a response to some particular item in the patient's environment, such as heights or confined spaces.

ADDers frequently develop a fear of socializing, particularly with large groups, and this is called a social phobia. This
problem may have resulted from the years of embarrassment
and humiliation caused by the patient's impulsivity, social
inappropriateness, and the subsequent peer rejection.

ADDers often report that public speaking is particularly
anxiety-provoking. One of our patients proclaimed that he
would rather "go ten rounds with Mike Tyson" than perform
any type of public speaking. He was an accomplished physician who was not only personally charming but extremely
witty in a private setting, but he became inordinately stiff and
sometime confused when called upon to address even small
groups of peers or patients. While treatment improved many
of this gentleman's symptoms, he never completely over-
came this phobic response.

Obsessive-Compulsive Disorder

In obsessive-compulsive disorder (OCD), individuals have
stereotypic thoughts, usually unpleasant. While obsessions
belong to the realm of thoughts, compulsions are actually ritu-
alistic, usually repetitive, nonpurposeful behaviors, such as
frequent washing of hands, checking repeatedly to see that the
coffee maker is turned off, and other compulsive behaviors.

These types of behavior are not commonly seen in attention deficit disorder, nor is OCD seen much as a co-morbidity.
However, in response to a lifetime of disorganization and
being a hostage to their unpredictable impulses, some adults

have developed certain self-policing traits to survive in the adult world. This "reactive paralysis" can transform banal, everyday-life decisions into existential deliberations.

Jennifer S. is a twenty-five-year-old woman who was seen in our clinic and received the diagnosis of attention deficit disorder after having to live with the consequences of poor choices.

> *Christmas was an absolute disastrous time for me every year. I would dread the holiday season for months in advance. However, this would not prompt me to begin my Christmas shopping earlier. . . . Hey, I have ADD! So, of course, I would wait until the very last minute to begin my shopping list, which was extremely long because I have always been so afraid of slighting someone. Often the gifts that I end up getting are very inappropriate and I have even offended friends and family members by my odd choices.*
>
> *Consequently, I report to the shopping mall more or less in a state of panic and go through the stores in my own harebrained manner. When I discover an item which I think might be right for one of my friends, I immediately become anxious. I try to second-guess the person's reaction to the gift and typically come up with some reason for not buying it.*
>
> *Invariably, after this several-hour, traumatic ritual, I come home empty-handed and then, when there is absolutely no time left, I report back to the mall, buy a bunch of stuff that no one will like, take the gifts home and then beat myself up over my silly choices. Merry Christmas.*

Personality Disorders

Personality is the aggregate of our emotional and behavioral traits that define and characterize us under routine circumstances. If one of these traits assumes "a life of its own" and dominates a person's personality, leading to impairment of functional ability and often personal distress, we say that the patient has a *personality disorder.* The overshadowing trait or behavior pattern is typically counterproductive in most spheres of living, pervasive, and virtually intolerable to the people in the sufferer's environment.

Such personality disorders are common; however, a complete review of all personality disorders is certainly beyond the scope of our discussion and only a few, ADD-relevant examples will be considered. Individuals with personality disorder have as defining characteristics hostility, rebelliousness, and an overall desire to get even. They frequently thrive on danger, self-promotion, and the misfortunes of others.

These traits are very similar to those seen in *oppositional defiant disorder* (ODD), which is seen in children. If the child's behavior is violent, the term *conduct disorder* (CD) is often invoked. One study reported in a 1993 issue of the *Archives of General Psychiatry* indicated that children carrying the diagnosis of attention deficit disorder had a ten times greater risk of developing antisocial personality disorder as adults than normal controls.

While this may represent the natural history of a subgroup of ADD, other environmental factors may also be at work in causing a personality disorder, such as extreme experiences of rejection, unusually rigid managing of the ADD symptoms by parents, and other factors. If the person with the personality disorder also had ADD, there is a risk multiplier for substance abuse.

Borderline Personality Disorder

Borderline personality disorder is another example of a condition that can mimic ADD for various reasons. Individuals suffering from this illness have a seriously disturbed self-image, as well as a poor relationship to their surroundings and erratic behavior with extreme fluctuations in mood. They can flip-flop from one emotional extreme to the other for reasons that mystify those around them. At one moment the individual may appear to be in a severe state of depression, but only moments later may be hostile, aggressive, or euphoric.

Brief psychotic episodes may occur with this behavior disorder. Individuals with borderline personality disorder are extremely unpredictable and are prone to self-mutilation (wrist slashing, etc.). They are very judgmental and regard every other human as either evil or saintly.

The resemblance to adult ADD is fairly superficial. Individuals with ADD are less rigid in their relationships to other human beings. The mood changes seen in ADD are usually traceable to an event in the individual's life, and self-destructive acts are infrequent. These individuals are incapable of empathy or involvement in an intimate relationship.

Substance Abuse

Individuals with undiagnosed ADD may have used and abused alcohol or other substances, including cocaine and marijuana. Often the basis for the dependence appears to be an attempt by the patient to self-medicate. Andrew G. was a patient in our ADD clinic, and gave us his story.

> I almost can't remember when I didn't drink. I began drinking in my early teens, usually when my parents were out of town. There were always large amounts of alcohol around the house and I could use this to impress my friends.
>
> As I have grown older, alcohol is not an amusement, but a necessity. When I come home from my job my mind is going a million miles a minute. I am dreaming up schemes for financial gain, as well as a thousand other projects. These thoughts and impulses are like ants crawling all over me.

> *As soon as I get home I begin drinking and finally the demons give me a break. In the mornings I have a different Satan to think about. I wake up every day with a serious hangover and am constantly late for work. I vow that this will be the last time but when I get home the demons are there waiting at the door like a devoted pet.*

Some individuals will abuse cocaine for the same purpose, and some use such over-the-counter medications as ephedrine. The behavioral patterns seen in someone abusing cocaine can be very similar to the symptoms seen in attention deficit disorder. Every physician treating ADD should ask about drug abuse.

Said Sam J., "After realizing I was fighting a losing battle against chemical dependency, I asked a friend for help. He sent me to be tested and bingo! I was diagnosed with ADHD." Now on medication, Sam is doing well, but he does has regrets over the past. "I feel that my ADHD led to substance abuse and also brought my marriage to an embarrassing and painful end."

Laura M. finds it particularly annoying that some doctors still believe that what people with ADD really want are stimulating medications. "I submit to them that if I wanted Dexedrine for kicks, I wouldn't be taking as little as I am. And if I were a speed addict, I wouldn't forget to take my medications as often!"

Sleep Disorders

Sleep disorders and attention deficit disorder share many common features. As with ADD, sleep disorders were typically treated by psychiatrists in the past. Psychiatric explanations of sleep disorders were stress, anxiety, altered mood, and sometimes work-related issues. But over the last two decades, increasing research has demonstrated a clear evidence of brain dysfunction in the person with a sleep disorder. As a result, sleep disorders and attention deficit disorder are both examples of the increasingly outmoded distinction between psychiatric illness and organic disease.

The *narcolepsy* syndrome is a fairly well-defined clinical entity which affects more than 100,000 individuals in the United States. The most striking symptom is the tendency for the individual to be sleepy during the day and actually fall asleep at inappropriate times—such as while driving, reading, and even while eating. Occasionally, these sleep attacks occur after ingestion of a meal rich in carbohydrates.

The sleep attacks can be quite irresistible and usually last less than thirty minutes, with up to eight sleep periods occurring in a single day. Beyond this excessive daytime somnolence pattern, these individuals suffer from cataplexy, which is one of the most fascinating disorders known to modern medicine.

Cataplexy, another symptom of narcolepsy, is a sudden loss of muscle tone and even paralysis, with the exception of the respiratory muscles. This usually affects the face, neck, and spine muscles, but can also affect the arms and legs. In severe attacks, individuals can actually fall and be injured. Typically, there is no alteration in the patient's awareness during these spells. Amazingly, these attacks of cataplexy can be provoked by laughter, anger, and virtually any emotion. Essentially any unexpected environmental stimulus can provoke an attack. Attacks can last from a few seconds to about ten minutes.

Difficulties with attention, task execution, remembering, and other ADD-like symptoms are well-described symptoms of narcolepsy. The distinction between attention deficit disorder and narcolepsy is based on a number of features, such as the presence of impulsivity, hyperactivity or inattention, and other features of ADD present since childhood.

Persons suffering from narcolepsy have a very characteristic blood abnormality, an abnormal marker molecule on their white blood cells. They also have an easily documented abnormality of sleep-related eye movements.

A more serious condition, *sleep apnea,* in most cases involves cessation of breathing while sleeping, usually based on an obstruction of the upper airways. While in mild cases this condition may result in mere excessive daytime sleepiness, sleep apnea can, in more extreme cases, lead to cardiac rhythm disturbances and even sudden death. The most typical complaint of this disorder will be drowsiness during the daytime with inappropriate falling-asleep, such as while driving, eating, or speaking.

Persons with this disorder also complain of difficulty focusing their attention, and poor performance at work. Changes in mood and personality are frequently seen in this disorder. The incidence of this disorder increases with age and approximately 90 percent of the sufferers are male.

The average age of onset is in the fifth decade of life, but has been reported in individuals in their early twenties. A distinction between sleep apnea and attention deficit disorder is usually fairly easy, based on the lack of attention deficit disorder-related symptoms in childhood, as compared to individuals with sleep apnea.

Other types of sleep disorders exist. Difficulty sleeping at night and sleep of poor quality can clearly interfere with function even of normal individuals. For this reason, it is extremely important for any physician treating attention deficit disorder to obtain an accurate and thorough history of the patient's nighttime sleeping habits and sensation of fatigue and sleepiness during the day as well.

Note: Be sure to read chapter 8 for some helpful hints on dealing with sleep disorders. Many people with ADD suffer from sleep disorders, although usually not as severe as the ones described in this chapter. If you suffer from insomnia or other common sleep problems, chapter 8 may help you.

II

Resolving the Problem

Now that we have defined the problem and given you an idea of whether you or someone you care about may have ADD, our next goal is to talk about practical solutions. First, you'll need to find a good physician, and we'll offer you important pointers to help lead you to an expert.

You'll also need to know about other therapies that can help, including medication, nonmedication forms of therapy, and unique new adaptive devices. And we don't want you to neglect your wellness quotient—many ADDers don't get enough sleep or exercise, and we have some solutions for you. All of these (and more) are our topics for Part II.

5

"Where Do I Start?"

After considering whether you may have some of the characteristics of ADD, the next step is to launch your "health quest," a journey to enhanced organization, attention, and improved interaction with others and to better health. But where do you start? As we discussed earlier, ADD is a neurobiological disorder and therefore it merits significant attention, treatment, and therapeutic intervention. In this chapter, we'll help you make a plan to find a good doctor and create and maintain a positive doctor-patient relationship.

"How Do I Choose a Doctor?"

Let's assume here that you do have attention deficit disorder and not one of the other medical problems that may mimic it. In this case, the first step you need to take is to ask your family doctor if he or she has any information on the problem. See how the doctor responds to your request. If, for example, your doctor states, "I think it is just a fad; other doctors just give out pills and build up their practice that way," then you'll need to seek help elsewhere. If, on the other hand, your doctor acknowledges ADD as a disorder, understands your concerns about having an ADD, and seems to have at least some basic knowledge about the disorder, then setting up an office visit with your doctor to discuss the issue may be appropriate.

The problem is that just as your Aunt Mary and Cousin Sally are influenced by negative press about ADD, so are many internists and general practitioners. (After all, doctors are people too.) There's also a lot of negative media surrounding medications, particularly central nervous system stimulants such as Ritalin and Dexedrine. As a result, many physicians are very reluctant to initiate an aggressive treatment regimen, which means that a lot of doctors may give you an extremely low and ineffectual dose of a stimulant and stop there.

Nevertheless, a good family physician who knows your background, your medical illnesses, and your personality may be invaluable in starting the diagnostic and treatment process.

"What If I Don't Have a Primary Care Doctor?"

What do you do if you don't have a family physician? You could look in the Yellow Pages, where you'll see all sorts of announcements and advertisements for physicians treating a variety of ailments. In fact, there even may be physicians specifically announcing they treat patients with attention deficit disorder. You *could* do this. But don't. Using the Yellow Pages alone as a way to select your doctor is a very bad idea because you have no way to gain a feel for what the doctor is like, how effective he is and how he treats patients.

Instead, we often recommend to our patients that they ask their friends if they've had experiences with a specific physician. If they have, and they say that they feel the doctor is very competent and they have a good rapport with this physician, then this certainly is high praise. Another way to locate a physician is through the local medical society, available in many communities. This organization can tell you about doctors accepting new patients. The downside with this tactic is that the medical society may not know if the doctor treats ADD.

An excellent starting point would be to contact the local ADD support group, particularly if the group includes adults who have ADD. We've listed names and organizations of support groups and therapists throughout the country in appendix III. Use this as a starting point to lead you to a local support group. For example, if the nearest group listed is a hundred miles away, call them and ask them if there are any groups for adults with ADD in your area.

You can also call Children and Adults with Attention Deficit Disorder (CH.A.D.D.), a national group and ask them for the nearest chapter. Although CH.A.D.D. doesn't differentiate adult ADD groups from groups that concentrate on children, it can still be helpful because even a group that devotes meetings to children is probably aware of the nearest adult ADD group.

Why We Think Neurologists Are Best

We are both board-certified neurologists, and because we believe that ADD is a neurologic disease, we also think that ADD is best diagnosed by a neurologist, particularly one interested in cognitive neurology.

Neurologists are medical doctors who treat a wide spectrum of disorders, from weakness and numbness, back pain, migraine headaches, spine disorders, stroke, seizures, convulsions, tremors, and other neurological ailments. They may also treat attention deficit disorder.

Most big cities and suburbs will have practicing neurologists available at medium to large hospitals, although if you live in a smaller community, you may need to travel to the nearest larger town or city to see a neurology specialist. The neurologist may be able to do the initial evaluation and outline a treatment plan for you, and if the distance is too far or terribly inconvenient for you, then the neurologist may be able to work in tandem with your local doctor. This option has worked well with some of our patients.

What About a Psychiatrist?

In the past and continuing into the present, psychiatrists have diagnosed and treated patients with ADD. In fact, the diagnosis of attention deficit disorder is actually outlined in the *Diagnostic and Statistical Manual IV (DSM-IV)*, routinely considered a psychiatric reference manual. Psychiatrists are very well trained to deal with disorders of behavior and mental illness, specifically as they have completed a training program in the social, psychological, and behavioral components of mental illness.

Over the last few years, psychiatric training programs have also strongly emphasized the biochemical and neurotransmitter role in psychiatric illness; we can see this emphasis in their use of a multitude of "traditional neurologic medications" such as antiseizure medicines for bipolar disorder (manic depression), as well as muscle relaxant medications for mood and anxiety disorders. We work very closely with our psychiatric colleagues, particularly to assess the behavioral component and to determine additional co-morbid features, which we discussed earlier.

In addition, as we've already noted, many different psychological and psychiatric disorders can manifest and appear as ADD, and these possibilities need to be ruled out. If other psychiatric problems are identified, then they are usually best treated by a psychiatrist. Psychiatrists are also medical doctors and thus they may prescribe medications.

While we like to tease our psychiatrist friends that "anyone who sees a psychiatrist should have his head examined," the reality is that in this day and age, psychiatric care is becoming more readily available and is also more widely covered by most major insurance carriers.

We still believe, however, that your first and best choice is to see a neurologist, because of the neurologist's very thorough background and comprehension of neurobiological disorders. In addition, many psychiatrists still concentrate on providing long-term therapy. It's also true that even though they may prescribe medications, some psychiatrists don't see medications as an important option—a viewpoint we don't share.

Some Simple Guidelines Before You See Your Doctor

Your doctor will help you determine if you have ADD, but it's a very good idea to plan ahead. Here are some simple suggestions to help you get the most from your visit with your physician.

1. Be prepared! This is important. The doctor-patient relationship is made up of two components, the doctor and you, the patient. If you come to the office visit on time, prepared to interact with the physician in a positive, yet assertive fashion, you'll be off to a good start.

   Come with a list of questions that you want to discuss at the time of the visit, as well as your specific concerns. The more specific you can be, the more your physician can address your questions. If, for example, you are certain you have ADD because you have met numerous criteria, and have already taken some of the basic questionnaires or tests (see appendix IV), bring them with you to your appointment. Usually, your physician will be glad to review these to determine if you are on the right track with your assessment of your disorder.

   Also, think ahead about general information the doctor will need, such as when you think your illness began, how it was diagnosed, how it has affected you, what you have done to adapt. It's also good to consider what things make your inattention and distractibility worse, and what things seem to help. (If you don't know, that's okay too.)

Remember, the doctor-patient relationship should be a positive experience, where you are both working to reach the same goal—your improved health. Being honest and forthright with your physician at the very onset will pay off in the future.

2. Make sure this doctor is comfortable treating patients with ADD or associated types of behavior and cognitive disturbances. Sadly, not every neurologist is. For example, you might want to ask the neurologist his opinion on the current thinking behind ADD, and if he responds, "Oh, I think children outgrow it when they reach adolescence," then look for a different doctor.

3. Ask the physician how many patients in the practice have a primary diagnosis of ADD. Does he seem current on and interested in ADD?

4. Ask the physician if she has both a short- and long-term treatment plan for ADD in general; for example, does she use medications, counseling, additional nonpharmacologic treatment? Or does she seem to believe that "Ritalin is the magic pill and that is all that I use"?

5. Ask the doctor if he has done any speaking engagements or work with local community chapters on ADD or other behavior disorders; this may give you a true insight into his degree of participation in this illness. For example, if the physician responds, "No, but I give a lot of seminars on spine pain," then you may have a glimpse into his true interest.

Also ask if he has done any background information or research into this topic. This certainly is fair game, as many neurologists have done research in their training or in their years after completion of training, and it would be helpful to find out what your physician's area of expertise really is.

More Thoughts on the Doctor-Patient Relationship

We feel that the doctor-patient relationship is very special, intimate, and also very delicate. When we deal with attention deficit disorder, we know that there are a lot of emotional, frustrating, and, at times, embarrassing issues that need to be discussed. In some ways, the doctor-patient relationship is like a marriage, and certainly this relationship can be critically important to your life. The physician's office can be likened to a bedroom in that it is very intimate and personal, and in that very important questions regarding your life, health, and future care will be discussed.

As in marriage, it's very important to be honest with your doctor and to feel that he or she is honest with you. If you feel uncomfortable in this relationship, it will be hard to communicate in an honest, open fashion and this will clearly inhibit your search for improved health.

In addition, be up front with your physician regarding what you are and are not willing to do with regard to your health care. For example, if finances limit expensive diagnostic testing, let your physician know that up front.

There are many ways to work out diagnostic testing and therapies on a payment plan, and just knowing that your physician is willing to work with you can make all the difference. In addition, sometimes there are research projects that are going on and you may be able to have diagnostic testing performed in a research fashion to defray some of the costs. If you can participate in a research project, then your treatment could be low-cost or free.

While we know that health care is expensive, ultimately the cost to a patient who is not treated is much more expensive. Poor job performance, lost wages, interpersonal strife, and marital failures take a significant toll on patients, particularly those who are unable or unwilling to receive treatment.

How You Feel About Medications Is Important, Too

Getting back to the issue of how far you are willing to go in terms of your health care, this is a cornerstone to your therapy. For example, if you are absolutely unwilling to take central nervous system stimulants, you must tell your physician that right at the onset. Conversely, if you have a specific goal to receive one of the of the centrally acting medications, such as Ritalin or Dexedrine, you should tell your physician that that is what you are expecting. This may not be what he or she is planning on prescribing, but at least your expectations will be laid out in an open fashion that you can both deal with.

One of us had a patient who presented himself for a diagnostic and therapeutic assessment following one of our ADD seminars. The patient said very adamantly, "I don't have a lot of money. I want to pay cash and I want to get medications to try." The patient assured me that he would try the medication and if he improved would proceed with all additional diagnostic testing. It's been over a year now, and the patient has refused further diagnostic testing. He says he feels "a little bit better" on the medications, and simply requests additional stimulant therapy.

This is an inappropriate way to proceed with treatment, and I told the patient so at the end of the year. He replied, "I don't want to have the rest of the testing. I guess I never really did, I just wanted to try the medications." This is distressing to a doctor and that type of dishonesty has led to a severed doctor-patient relationship.

If there are therapies, treatments, or tests with which you know you have absolutely no way to comply, nor have any intention of complying, please inform your physician as the plan is made. It looks silly in the medical record to have a physician outlining a plan with A, B, C, and D as components, when you know you will do none of them. Ultimately, that visit and therapeutic recommendation are not only a waste of the physician's time, but a waste of your finances.

Doctors Are Human, Too

No matter which type of physician you see as an assessment for your disorder, please don't forget that physicians are humans, not gods. Although the physician has spent many years in education and training, she's not a psychic and can't read your mind. You must be able to communicate effectively, which is something we stress repeatedly at our seminars and educational conferences.

We will often start our conferences with a slide showing a man in a sand trap playing golf, looking up at his wife saying, "hand me a sand wedge"; the wife reaches down and hands him a sandwich. If this is the type of communication you are receiving, or even if you feel you are communicating as best as you are able and this is the response you are getting, it may be time to move on to obtain an additional opinion.

Working together collaboratively, you and your physician should be able to shed a new light onto your diagnosis, as well as open many new avenues for treatment options. Working together mountains can be moved or, as the saying goes, "Out of chaos, order."

Evaluating a Prospective Physician for Yourself

What else will determine if you are going to have a successful relationship with your physician?

1. Promptness is important. If your physician is late, and you are constantly on time (or vice versa), this may be a poor match for you.

2. What is the staff like? If the staff treats you as you would want to be treated, with courtesy and attention, then this is certainly a positive sign. If the first question is, "How are you going to pay?", that is an indication of the staff and physician's priorities.

While certain questions are delicate and difficult and by necessity need to be answered, there is always the appropriate way to have this information presented, with hopefully a wide range of acceptable answers.

If the staff appears rigid, inflexible, and uncompromising, you can expect that you will have the same result when you call in for questions or problems. On the other hand, if the staff is quite interested in obtaining additional medical records, obtaining any additional testing, reports, etc., that may be helpful in making a diagnosis, then you can see how the physician and his staff's priorities lie.

3. What is the office policy? Is there a stated office policy? Is there a specific billing policy, and what is expected up front? Will the physician bill your insurance provider? Are you expected to pay half, or pay the complete bill at the time of the visit? What if finances are a hardship? Will the physician's billing manager arrange a payment plan? These are certainly very reasonable questions to ask, and do not be embarrassed about doing so.

If you have been referred to a specific physician by a friend who thinks this doctor is "the greatest," keep in mind that every patient and every personality brings something different to the doctor-patient relationship. What one individual finds promising, exciting, and therapeutic, another may find distasteful or unpleasant. We encourage our patients to be the best patient they can be—that is, to be prepared, be present, approach the relationship with a positive outlook—and we feel that we will have something to offer every individual.

The bottom line is that this is your health care and, of course, health care is a precious resource indeed. You need to investigate it even more thoroughly than you would investigate the purchase of any new vehicle or appliance. This is one area where you should work hard to restrain your impulsivity and seriously consider the pros and cons of an individual physician.

It is also important that you have a good doctor whom you can work with *because of* the ADD. Adults with attention deficit disorder are disorganized and scattered enough without imposing additional obstacles of an unfriendly or inflexible office staff or physician. It is important to get started, but getting started in the right direction may make all the difference in helping you obtain your goals.

Psychologists

Psychologists are mental health professionals who have trained for a number of years, receiving their Ph.D. in psychology. Many patients confuse psychologists and psychiatrists. Psychologists do not prescribe medications and are not medical doctors. *Psychiatrists* are medical doctors and can prescribe medications.

Although they cannot write you a prescription, many psychologists are extremely skilled in counseling. Often they specialize in various aspects of behavior, such as behavior modification, biofeedback, hypnotherapy, and/or relaxation techniques. They are often very skilled in dealing with the emotional and psychological issues that are secondary to this disorder.

We work very closely with a number of psychologists, particularly in allowing the psychologist to do the paper and pencil testing of ADD—often very helpful in terms of making an accurate diagnosis—as well as in determining the severity of impairment, associated with this disorder.

While a one- or two-page screening test can be done quickly in the office by any family physician or professional, psychologists will often complete a battery of cognitive and behavioral tests that can truly identify which parts of the brain are functioning efficiently, which parts are functioning slightly less so, and which parts are functioning poorly if at all.

Many of these professionals are also very skilled with cognitive retraining; that is, using adaptive devices, including computer programs, to retrain the brain to think in a more logical and organized fashion. We discus this in further detail in chapter 9, on technology, as well as in chapter 7, on other treatment therapies.

6

Medications

───⌐⊶⊷⊶⊷⌐───

Canadian physician Sir William Osler once said, "The desire to take medication is perhaps the greatest feature that separates man from animals." We believe, however, that it is actually the desire to be well and to maintain as normal a lifestyle as possible that drives our patients to seek not only medical assistance, but also appropriate medication for their attention deficit disorder.

This chapter will delve into the various types of medications that are useful and effective for treatment of adults with attention deficit disorder. We will start out by talking about the cornerstone of therapy, the central nervous system stimulants. Then we'll move on to medications that fall into the class called *antidepressant agents* but which are also truly effective in affecting the central nervous system chemical messengers of the brain—and hence, helping the person with ADD.

In addition, there are classes of medications such as those routinely used for blood pressure, those used for movement disorders and even for seizure disorders that are now finding new uses in attention deficit disorder. We will also briefly discuss some new medicines on the horizon. And we will explain why many individuals need more than one medication to treat their ADD.

It's important to note that dosages must be adjusted to individual needs, starting with the lowest possible dose and increasing to an efficacious level. Some physicians, fearing abuse potential of stimulant medications, have underprescribed such medications as Ritalin or Dexedrine, despite the fact that there appears to be little abuse potential among those who have attention deficit disorder.

One problem we've noticed is that the popular media have made it virtually impossible for patients to feel comfortable about taking medication for this disorder. "If you would just pull yourself together," they seem to say, "you would do just fine." This fundamental lack of knowledge and understanding by the general population makes this disorder quite frustrating to deal with. Patients are reluctant and sometimes even loath to seek medical attention because of the stigma attached to ADD. In addition, the environment can be difficult for physicians eager to help people with ADD with what modern science and technology has to offer today.

Sometimes the negative press about medications for ADD can be nearly unbelievable to doctors today. To show you what we mean, imagine the following information that we've written in the style of popular media hysteria-speak.

From 1994 to 1995, sales of Humulin have increased from $665 million to $794 million! This means a 19 percent surge in sales for the producers of this type of genetically engineered insulin. Does this mean that our people are being drugged out with a dangerous, trendy new drug? Can this be the latest fad doctors are trying out, egged on by the desire to try the latest and greatest? Are people signing up for this drug without seriously considering the consequences?

And there's more! Statistics show that the number
of patients with insulin-dependent diabetes mellitus has
been increasing year by year. But nearly 60 percent of
the population with diabetes is undiagnosed and
untreated. Is this due to inadequate medical knowl-
edge? Could this be due to health care changes? Are
people unable to gain access into the health care sys-
tem? Someone should investigate!

The above is an illustration of the ridiculous way the media
has treated attention deficit disorder—except we substituted
diabetes for ADD and Humulin for Ritalin. Certainly, no physician worth his license would prescribe insulin to a patient if
that was not the medication of choice, and Humulin is a good
medication for many patients with this form of diabetes. Nor
would a good doctor withhold medication from patients who
need it.

Now look at what the popular press has said about Ritalin
and other medications prescribed for ADD. They wonder
aloud if medication usages have skyrocketed unreasonably.
They agonize over whether this is just the latest fad that doctors have latched on to. They postulate that maybe doctors
are giving too many people too many (and too high of a
dosage) of these medications. And they criticize the pharmaceutical companies who produce medications for ADD.

The point is, with any medical situation the least invasive
therapy is always the best. You don't do brain surgery if a person has a migraine, nor do you put that person on narcotics if
Tylenol would work. As a result, the least amount of medication that works is always the most appropriate dosage.

When it comes to insulin-dependent diabetics, if this
medication were withheld, one could imagine the consequences: seizures, diabetic coma, severe nerve damage,
heart disease, heart attacks, strokes, and ultimately death.
Certainly this is a serious medical issue and is also why doctors are eager to identify a patient who has diabetes mellitus,
treat the patient appropriately, and follow that patient closely

to make sure the treatment stays appropriate throughout the course of therapy.

Many People with ADD Need Medication

The illustration of the individual with insulin-dependent diabetes mellitus who needs Humulin (or other medication) closely parallels the situation of the patient with attention deficit disorder. ADD is a true neurobiological and chemical disorder requiring not only counseling, therapy, hand-holding, and reassurance, but also our patients with this disorder frequently require the use of medications. They need to replace the chemicals in their brains that are deficient. If they don't receive the chemicals they need, then their behavior and their overall lives will be impaired.

Therefore, we think it is ridiculous that the popular press has made a target of Ritalin, one of the foundation medications of treatment for attention deficit disorder. Study after study has shown that this is an effective therapy. And, as every one of our patients who has succeeded with Ritalin can attest, their function, both on a cognitive level (that is, scoring higher on standardized tests) as well as on a social, interpersonal, and general behavior level is markedly improved by the medication.

It is true, as a number of studies have pointed out, that individuals with attention deficit disorder seem to have very minimal addictive qualities to these medications. But people with ADD often gain a significant positive response in terms of their ability to function in normal, everyday activities. Just as Humulin, a synthetic insulin, is an effective and appropriate therapy for individuals with diabetes, so are the multitude of medications available today for attention deficit disorder effective and appropriate therapies for this disease.

We think that, from an ethical standpoint, it is not only inhumane, but cruel and unusual to withhold medications for an illness that can so readily be treated, simply because the popular press is ignorant of this disorder, despite the great wealth of research and literature available today on the success of medications for ADD.

One other important comment should be related to our analogy of treating insulin dependent diabetics versus treating patients with attention deficit disorder. Lilly, the drug company that has a significant interest in insulin production and distribution, posted significant fourth-quarter earnings per share of 57 cents in 1995, an increase of 21 percent. Likewise, Ciba-Geigy, the makers of Ritalin, have made a significant profit, as there has been a steadily increasing demand for the medication dating back to 1990, with demand outstripping the supply over the last few years.

But while the popular press has maligned Ciba-Geigy for making Ritalin, a medication that is increasing in popularity and use, inciting corporate profits as the reason to "rein in this company," no one is criticizing Lilly. Nor should they.

These two corporations, and other pharmaceutical companies like them, serve a key function—to perform the research and development to identify and produce and sell the chemicals that have a positive impact on patients' lives. Usage for both these medications is going up, but we believe that is proof in itself that the medications are effective and provide a positive benefit for the patients who take them. Clearly, if the medication was ineffective, sales would plummet and the pharmaceutical companies would rethink whether it should be sold.

The Central Nervous System Stimulants

Reaching for Ritalin

Ritalin is truly one of the cornerstones of therapy for attention deficit disorder. Its main psychoactive chemical, known as methylphenidate hydrochloride, is chemically a central nervous system stimulant. How does it work? As outlined in the *Physicians' Desk Reference*, its mechanism of action is not entirely understood. Researchers think that it activates the brain stem, particularly what is known as the arousal system (ascending reticular activating system).

In effect, by turning up the volume of brain stimulation, Ritalin can actually produce its stimulant effect. By increasing the stimulation of the arousal or attention center of the nervous system, the medication increases or stimulates the filtering system, thus allowing individuals to focus on specific issues rather than trying to attend to everything.

In chapter 2, where we discussed various theories of ADD's causes, we mentioned the theory that the brain's filter is simply not working correctly, and too much information is being processed all at once, thus a lot of important information falls through. Ritalin can apparently produce a more effective sieve, allowing individuals to attend to the appropriate stimuli and let the irrelevant slide on through, rather than attending to multiple stimuli. As a result, patients can focus and be less easily distracted.

The doctor's goal in prescribing this medicine is to improve your attention, alertness, memory, and concentration. By doing so, it also often has a secondary positive effect of reducing behavior problems, social problems, impulsivity, and certainly has, in our experience, reduced the potential for "acting out" (throwing adult-sized temper tantrums).

Susan K., who was diagnosed with ADD at the age of twenty-three, after enduring a very difficult struggle through college, said, "When I took Ritalin for the first time, I thought, no wonder people do well in school—they have this super power I never had. I looked back at the way I would marvel at students studying for hours at a time, not fidgeting, getting up, daydreaming, or driving themselves crazy. It was indeed a power!"

Ritalin is provided as tablets of 5, 10, and 20 mg, and is taken by mouth. In addition, there is a long-acting "sustained release" (SR) tablet of 20 mg that need not be taken as frequently. The regular tablets are relatively quick-acting, getting into your system within about 30 minutes, in our experience. Their effects last from 3 to 4 hours (although, as with any medication, each person's response is unique).

Ritalin dosage can be varied somewhat, depending on the individual's needs. For example, if you absolutely must be attentive in the early morning and midday, but it's all right if you are less attentive in the evening, then your dosage could be adjusted and timed so that the maximum dose would affect you in the early morning and midday and you would receive a lower dose (or no dose) for later during the day.

People with ADD usually avoid taking Ritalin four to six hours prior to bedtime, because it can produce insomnia.

How long Ritalin SR will benefit you varies, and ranges anywhere from 6 to 8 hours, although again this length of action varies from individual to individual. The SR 20 mg dosage has the same side effects and beneficial effect profiles as the standard shorter-acting medication. The primary benefit for many people is that it's more convenient. In addition, as many sufferers of this disorder are painfully aware, remembering to take medications is often a tricky issue; anything that can be done that makes medication adjustment or management less complex, or that allows the patient to be more compliant with dosing, is certainly worthwhile.

How much Ritalin is enough? Interestingly, the dosage regimen, as listed in the *Physicians' Desk Reference*, lists 40 to 60 mg daily, though it acknowledges that other individuals may respond to a significantly lesser dose, and an "average dose is 20–30 mg daily." A recent article in the January 1996 issue of *Southern Medical Journal* suggests this dosing scheme may lead to partial success. On the other hand, it may also explain the significant failure rate for individuals taking this medication. What they may have needed was a higher dose of the medication.

As a matter of fact, the study revealed there was a 97-percent success rate using stimulants when the medication was pushed up until the person reached a therapeutic benefit.

The upper limit was determined by either (a) improvement of symptoms to the point that no further medication adjustment was needed, or (b) side effects, as listed above, that became intolerable or unacceptable.

With this dosage scheme, moderately more liberal than that recommended in the *Physicians' Desk Reference,* it was easier for these physicians to obtain a significantly higher success rate than many physicians experienced using this medication at lower doses.

Physicians are allowed to use any medication on an individual basis with a patient, titrating the dosage to achieve the maximal benefit and minimal side effects.

A *transdermal* (through the skin) form of Ritalin is in the works. This is not yet available for use in the United States.

Stimulant Medications Can Have Side Effects

All of the medications in this class of central nervous system stimulants have a similar side-effects profile that could include any or all of the following: nervousness, irritability, insomnia, edginess, anorexia, weight loss, slight tremor, blood pressure elevation, mood swings and dysphoria, headaches and, in rare cases, seizure.

There has been a significant debate in neurologic literature as to whether Ritalin truly produces a tic or involuntary movement disorders. We think that a high enough dosage of this medication can actually unmask a latent or hidden tic disorder, but is not responsible in and of itself for producing that disorder. However, this aspect is relatively controversial, and the final word about motor tics is uncertain.

Dexedrine (dextroamphetamine)

Dexedrine is also in the class of central nervous system stimulants, and is another quite popular and relatively effective medication for treatment of adults with attention deficit disorder.

Dexedrine is an amphetamine and consequently has a risk potential for abuse. And, of course, any type of central nervous system medication needs to be carefully monitored.

Dexedrine comes in short-acting tablets of 5 mg or longer-acting "spansule" time-release capsules of a 5, 10, or 15 mg dosage. Their mechanism of action is fairly similar to that of Ritalin with all of the same positive effects, as well as the risk for many of the same adverse effects.

A spansule is like a capsule. It usually contains miniballs of medication, and the inside of each ball is coated differently and therefore is dissolved or absorbed at various times, thus giving you your delayed and prolonged medication effect.

These medications have also been known to produce some moderate weight loss, and have been labeled "anorectics." This does *not* mean that Dexedrine is a good medication to take if you need to lose a few pounds. You should only take medication you need, and if you do not have ADD, then you *don't* need Dexedrine.

Dexedrine can interact with many other medications and therefore it is mandatory that any physician prescribing these medications have a clear knowledge and understanding of any additional medications that you may be on. The problem is that Dexedrine (or any other medications in this class) can either increase or completely block the effects of other medications you may be taking. Be sure to report all medications you take to your doctor, including any over-the-counter medications such as cold medicine, and even vitamins.

Adderall

A third medication in this class is Adderall, previously known as Obetrol. Adderall was initially promoted as a medication for weight loss, but it later became known that it could be effective in treating ADD as well.

Adderall has received a lot of attention on the Internet, in popular literature, and amongst some physicians. But we are uncertain that there is any specific benefit of this medication over the more traditional Ritalin or even Dexedrine. Certainly, long-term prospective studies would be helpful in determining which of these three medications have the most beneficial effect and with the least degree of adverse side effects.

Cylert

Another very popular medication in the treatment of attention deficit disorder is *Cylert* (pemoline). While this medication is a central nervous system stimulant, its chemical makeup and structure is somewhat different from Ritalin, Dexedrine, and Adderall.

Cylert is supplied as tablets in a peculiar dosage, 18.75 mg, 37.5 mg, and 75 mg. It is also available as a chewable tablet containing 37.5 mg. As with other central nervous system stimulants, it is not entirely clear how this medication works. Some experts believe that Cylert stimulates the dopamine system. (For more information, read chapter 2 on causes of ADD.) But the exact site, location, and mechanism of action is not known.

Cylert does have some differences from the other central nervous system stimulants. This medication seems to be less addicting or habit-forming compared to the other stimulant medications. Its onset of action is somewhat slower, usually having a peak onset of action within 2 to 4 hours of taking the medication, lasting anywhere from 6 to 8 hours in the bloodstream.

As a result, if you need to pay attention soon, for example, at school, business, or executive meetings, keep in mind that this medication has a slower onset but longer duration of action. Also, if there is any type of negative effect, this may take longer to remove itself from the bloodstream, as compared to the other medications.

One note of caution: Cylert is metabolized through the liver and requires careful liver monitoring. It is essential to pick up any liver dysfunction early so the medication can be stopped and appropriate actions can be taken.

For some reason, Cylert does not seem to carry the negative stigma that Ritalin carries and, indeed, many individuals prefer to take this medication because it is less well recognized by the general population.

Cocaine

Although cocaine is an illegal drug when sold on the streets (and a drug that can be prescribed by doctors for some conditions), it would be an oversight to ignore its impact when discussing the effects of medications on the central nervous system. Cocaine is available as a prescription medication for some uses but is not used for ADD. Cocaine works on a particular part of the dopamine system pathways that carry dopamine, causing rapid stimulation of specific parts of the brain. It is this rapid change that seems to produce the cocaine high, rather than the specific site where the medication acts.

People with ADD who have experimented with cocaine illegally have reported that they do not get the high, but rather are more clearly organized, more alert, less impulsive, and more attentive. However, they state that cocaine is not as beneficial as some of the more traditional central nervous system stimulants.

Cocaine produces stimulation for a short period of time, but then wears off quickly. Ritalin, Dexedrine, and Cylert all produce improved attention, organized thought, less impulsivity for longer periods of time, and have a more gradual wearing off effect than does cocaine.

Some say that the Native Americans who chewed on the cocoa plant had less of a high and less addiction potential than contemporary individuals who smoke or freebase cocaine, as the chewing effect slows the onset. People who have experimented with cocaine do *not* prefer that chemical over the more traditional central nervous system stimulants, pointing out that the more traditional medications work better and longer.

The Tricyclic Antidepressant Medications

There are other medications that are effective for individuals with attention deficit disorder and work on the brain, brain chemical pathways, and central nervous system. One class of medications that can be effective in treating ADD are the tricyclic antidepressants. Some examples of tricyclic antidepressants are *Tofranil* (imipramine) and *Elavil* (amitriptyline), *Pamelor* (nortriptyline), and *Norpramin* (desipramine).

These medications, when they work, enhance the brain's filtering function and consequently improve attention, memory, organization, and thought. In addition, these antidepressant medications, as their name implies, are often quite helpful for treating a common secondary aspect of this disorder, major depression itself. Depression is common among people with ADD, and tricyclic antidepressants seem to be more effective than are the central nervous system stimulants in treating and improving patients who suffer from both depression and ADD.

These medications come in various tablets, ranging from 10 mg all the way up to 100 mg. The usual dosage regimen is a slow and steadily increasing dosage of the medication. Your doctor should carefully monitor side effects and allow enough time for the medication to fully benefit you.

Don't expect immediate results, but do expect some improvement within two to three weeks. You may experience some side effects in the first few days. Side effects range from nervousness, fatigue, insomnia, sleep cycle derangement, gastrointestinal distress, and dizziness, to blood pressure changes, accelerated heart rate and, on rare occasions, heart rhythm disturbances.

In addition, most of these medications produce some degree of dry mouth, and sometimes blurred vision. Men may have trouble urinating. Men with any degree of prostate problems should discuss this with your physician prior to initiating these medications. Anyone with any type of cardiac disorder or heart rhythm disturbance should clearly make sure that the doctor is fully aware of this before prescribing this medication.

The onset of action is highly variable, but most of the tricyclics will stay in the bloodstream at least twenty-four hours and in some cases much longer. These medications should never be discontinued without the full and complete consent of your personal physician. A sudden withdrawal can cause a rebound effect, and can actually trigger many of the medical side effects discussed.

Monoamine Oxidase Inhibitors

Eldepryl (deprenyl, selegiline HCL) A monoamine oxidase (MAO) inhibitor is most commonly used in the treatment of Parkinson's disease. Its chemical action is not completely understood, but the medication has an effect on the membranes of mitochondria, the cells' energy powerhouses in our body. The monoamine oxidase has the important role of breaking down stress chemicals (catecholamines) that include such chemical agents as dopamine, norepinephrine, epinephrine, and serotonin. When these scavengers (MAOs) are blocked, the chemicals that would have normally been destroyed remain in the brain tissue and throughout the body for longer periods of time.

One problem is that although higher levels of dopamine (as well as norepinephrine and serotonin) are all very important for many processes in the brain—including improved thought and intention—the MAO inhibitor can often produce significant side effects. The more serious side effects of this medication include hypertensive crisis (severe critical elevated high blood pressure), palpitations, hyperpyrexia (severe increase in body temperature), and even, on rare occasions, death.

Lesser side effects can include a dry mouth, occasional involuntary movements, leg pains, muscle cramps, joint aching, hair loss, and malaise.

Eldepryl comes as a 5 mg tablet and dosage is suggested to be limited to 10 mg per day because at a higher dosage, it may precipitate negative side effects in some individuals.

Although there are studies outlining the use of deprenyl in attention deficit disorder, we do not use this as a first line of therapy; however, one study indicated that deprenyl was effective in the treatment of children with Tourette's syndrome who also had attention deficit disorder. A large number of people with Tourette's—perhaps as many as 70 percent—also have ADD. Many people with Tourette's experience a worsening of their tics and other symptoms when they take such drugs as Ritalin, thus deprenyl may be a possible alternative after more study is made on both children and adults.

Nevertheless, we have had extensive experience with this medication in our patients with Parkinson's disease. It's also true that an additional role for benefit in Parkinson's includes a presumed antioxidant, neuroprotective effect. We are uncertain if this could play a positive role in individual attention deficit disorder.

Selective Serotonin Reuptake Inhibitors (SSRIs)

This class of antidepressant medication truly hit its stride in the 1990s with the original serotonin reuptake inhibitor of Prozac, (fluoxetine HCL). This medication was an original, chemically unrelated to any of the prior antidepressant medications. The chemical in Prozac can work as an antidepressant and also has an anti-obsessive/compulsive action. Experts believe that it blocks the reuptake of serotonin, one of the chemical messengers of the brain. As a result, there is more serotonin in the central nervous system and it is available longer.

The medication is supplied as *pulvules* (similar to spansules) of 10 and 20 mg, as well as oral/liquid 20 mg/5 ml, mint flavor elixir. Prozac seems to have a peak onset of action at approximately 6 to 8 hours after initial dosage. The full positive effect of the medication may take up to fourteen to twenty-one days, although adverse reactions may be seen over the first series of days.

Side effects that have been noted include a slight increase in anxiety, nervousness, and sleep dysfunction. Insomnia has been noted. Drowsiness and/or fatigue, sensation of restlessness, or tremor has been noted. There have been some complaints of gastrointestinal distress, as well as anorexia, some nausea, and dizziness. Most of these side effects are fairly short-lived.

Prozac was originally outlined for treatment of depression and obsessive/compulsive disorders, but we have also found it to be effective for some patients with ADD as well as extremely effective in patients who suffer from migraine headaches. (See our book, *Migraine—What Works!*)

We find that a dosage of anywhere from 10 up to 80 mg has been effective, and every individual responds in a unique way to this medication. In addition, as we have mentioned with other antidepressant medications, patients seem to respond quite well to this medicine when there is a co-morbid aspect of depression and anxiety.

Other Selective Serotonin Reuptake Inhibitors (SSRIs)

There are also other very powerful medications in this same class, including *Paxil* (paroxetine), *Zoloft* (sertraline), and a recent addition, *Luvox* (fluvoxamine). While these are all selective serotonin reuptake inhibitors, they all have a slightly different mechanism of action and all have a slightly different response profile.

Paxil (paroxetine HCL)   *Paxil* is available as 20 mg pink scored tablets, 30 mg blue tablets, with a recommended initial dose of 20 mg per day. Dosages may be increased in increments of 10 mg per week. Again, the onset of action and duration until therapeutic benefit may take a series of days to a few weeks.

The multiple side effects noted are quite similar to those found with Prozac. Many of our patients who show minimal response to Prozac have responded nicely to Paxil. Therefore, just because one medication in a class of medications has not worked that does not mean that other medicines in that same class will not be successful.

Zoloft (sertraline HCL)   *Zoloft* is yet another serotonin reuptake inhibitor quite similar to Prozac and Paxil. At steady state, it appears as though peak dose of activity occurs between 4.5 and 8.5 hours following medication initiation.

According to the *Physicians' Desk Reference,* Zoloft's half-life elimination is approximately 26 hours. The *half-life* is the time for a medicine (when it is at a steady state) to be half eliminated from the body, so that only half is left. The longer the half-life, the longer the positive or negative effects will last. Therefore, there appears to be longer action of this medication as compared to some of the other medications.

Zoloft comes as 50 mg tablets in a light blue film-coated tablet, scored, as well as 50 and 100 mg scored, capsule-shaped tablets. The benefit and side effect profile is very similar to the other serotonin reuptake inhibitor medications.

Luvox (fluvoxamine maleate)   This serotonin reuptake inhibitor is slightly chemically different than the SSRIs mentioned above, and therefore warrants additional mention. *Luvox* comes as 50 and 100 mg tablets. After steady state is reached, the peak dose after medication consumption is 3 to 8 hours.

One additional tablet can actually cause much higher blood level dosing than would be expected, as the more medication one takes, the quicker the rise in the serum bloodstream of this chemical.

This medication has the standard side effects as the other serotonin reuptake inhibitors, including general malaise, headaches, palpitations, nausea, stomach upset, diarrhea, and vomiting, as well as sleep dysfunction, nervousness, anxiety, and sometimes tremor.

Because Luvox is a newer medication, it is unclear if complete positive benefit and complete side effect profile is as thoroughly established and recognized as some of the other serotonin reuptake inhibitors. Nevertheless, we have had patients who have responded very nicely to this medication and it is certainly reasonable to prescribe it.

Atypical Antidepressant Agents

Wellbutrin (bupropion HCL)   *Wellbutrin* is significantly different from the other antidepressant medicines we have discussed previously. It appears to be a relatively weak blocker of reuptake of serotonin and norepinephrine. It seems to inhibit the reuptake of dopamine to some extent. Animal studies have shown this medication does produce dose-related effects in the form of stimulation, but extremely high doses have been known to produce negative side effects.

This medication is supplied as tablets of 75 and 100 mg, and appears to have a relatively weak onset of action within two hours, after steady state is achieved, with a range of half-life anywhere from 8 to 24 hours.

Wellbutrin has been used as an antidepressant with a stimulating effect, and many patients have experienced positive results. Some interesting studies of this medication in its use for attention stimulation and attention deficit disorder document the positive role that Wellbutrin can play in individuals with ADD.

This medication has the standard list of adverse effects seen in some of the medications we have previously discussed, including heart rhythm disturbance, blood pressure

changes, dizziness, appetite changes, weight changes, gastrointestinal distress, as well as a sense of restlessness, agitation, anxiety, and confusion. We have also seen the side
effects of dry mouth, irritability, and a sensation of mild confusion, all of which seem to improve over a series of days.
Again, as with many of the other centrally acting medications, it may take anywhere from ten to twenty-one days for
this medication to have its positive effect.

Although the recommended medication dosage is 300 mg
per day, we have had some good response using a slightly
lower dosage and, indeed, have very slowly and steadily
increased this medication up to a maximum of 300 mg per day.[1]

Serzone (nefazodone HCL)   *Serzone,* like bupropion in Wellbutrin, is also unrelated to the prior standard antidepressant
medicines. It does not have a chemical structure similar to the
serotonin reuptake inhibitors, or to the tricyclic, tetracyclic, or
monoamine oxidase inhibitor medications. As with most of the
other medications, its direct mechanism of action is unknown.
It seems to work on the central nervous system, having moderate effect on serotonin and norepinephrine in the brain tissue.

The medication comes in a multitude of dosages, including
100, 150, 200, and 250 mg tablets. It has a relatively rapid onset
of action with peak concentrations of the medication at approximately one hour with half-life ranging from 2 to 4 hours.

While the *Physicians' Desk Reference* lists this medication
as indicated for the treatment of depression, we are very
excited about its use in individuals with attention deficit disorder. Long-term studies involving this medication have not yet
been performed, as it is still relatively new, but we have seen a
positive impact in our patients who initially sought treatment
for depression and who also have attention deficit disorder.

As with other medications that work on the central nervous system, Serzone has the standard list of side effects,

---

1. FDA approval is being sought for a sustained-release (longer-acting) form of
   Wellbutrin.

ranging from headache, nausea, diarrhea, and constipation, to more significant symptoms of lightheadedness and low blood pressure, postural blood pressure changes, confusion, and memory impairment. However, the more common side effects with this medication appear to be initially sleepiness or, in some individuals, altered sleep cycle, stomach upset, and dry mouth.

Serzone has a slightly more complex dosing regimen, as evidenced by the multiple dosages it comes in. The recommended starting dose is 200 mg per day, although we have found that by starting at a slightly lower dose, 100 mg per day, we have avoided many of the negative side effects. Serzone is relatively easy to titrate up in increments of 100 mg per day, with many of our patients responding to a dose of 300 to 400 mg per day. We did see fewer negative side effects in individuals who were on lower dosages.

We feel that Serzone holds great promise, not only for its antidepressant effect, but also for its positive stimulant effects and cognitive effects in our patients.

Dopamine Agonists

As we outlined in chapter 2, on various theories about the causes of ADD, the role of dopamine, the dopamine receptors, and chemical interactions of the brain with the dopamine pathway seem to play a very significant role in attention deficit disorder. Therefore, it is not surprising that agents that stimulate the dopamine system would have a profound effect on individuals with ADD.

Parlodel (bromocriptine mesylate) *Parlodel* is a very potent dopamine receptor *agonist.* That means that it stimulates the receptor that dopamine works on, making this a much more effective receptor. The medication comes as either 2.5 mg or 5.0 mg. Parlodel seems to not only work on the dopamine system but also have an effect on the pituitary gland, and inhibits the release of the chemical prolactin.

Parlodel seems to have a stronger role in neurology in patients with Parkinson's disease, and is considered a very effective adjunct treatment to other therapies for Parkinson's. In addition, more standard uses for this medication include disorders of the pituitary gland, particularly disorders of excess secretion of prolactin. However, there have been studies of this dopamine agonist and its effect on cognition and attention; for this reason it is included in this discussion of prescription medications.

Multiple side effects are noted with the use of Parlodel, including lightheadedness, faintness, some nausea and vomiting, stiffness, excess movements, appetite suppression, headache, fatigue, with rare findings of elevated liver functions. While Parlodel is not considered a primary therapeutic medication for attention deficit disorder, there have been some studies on its effectiveness; the exact long-term role of this medication in ADD, however, is uncertain.

Antihypertensive Medications

Antihypertensives are made to lower the body's blood pressure. However, they also seem to lower the sympathetic outflow, or the "fight or flight" nervous system response. By toning down the stress chemicals in the body, there seems to be an accompanying general organization of thought and attention, and in this way antihypertensive medications may have the paradoxical effect of improving individuals' concentration and attention with this disorder.

Beta Blockers Beta blockers are traditionally used as a blood pressure medication, but are also widely used in neurology for migraine headache prevention. There are numerous medications in this category. The most commonly used and well known is Inderal, and the generic form of this is propranolol. This medication comes in 10, 20, 40, 60, 80, 120, and 160 mg dosages. As mentioned, these medications have a direct effect on the sympathetic nervous system, described specifically as a nonselective beta adrenergic receptor block-ing agent. (See our book, *Migraine—What Works!*)

There are a number of warnings that need to be followed if you are taking a beta blocker, particularly for individuals with significant heart disease. Anyone with a respiratory dis-turbance (particularly asthma) or upper airway disease should avoid this medication.

We have had a great deal of experience with Inderal and its multiple cousins under different trade names, particularly for blood pressure, migraine, and for essential tremor. While there is a wide variety of side effects, of which the most com-mon we deal with include low blood pressure, slow pulse, fatigue, hair loss and, in men, on rare occasions, generalized mild decrease in libido and sexual performance.

This medication may have a significant role in co-phar-macy (using two drugs to treat a specific disorder) and, specifi-cally, in comanaging patients who have side effects of more traditional medications such as Ritalin and some of the antide-pressants described earlier. For example, if the stimulant med-ications are helpful, but they cause increased blood pressure or tremor, then adding a second medication such as Inderal would allow the patient to continue taking the stimulant.

Catapres (clonidine HCL)   This medication is a very promi-nent antihypertensive medication. It is available as both an oral tablet and as a patch. Catapres has also gained wide popularity in the treatment of attention deficit disorder in children.

While its approved use is in the role of blood pressure regulation, its mechanism of action seems to stimulate cer-tain receptors in the brain stem, resulting in essentially a ton-ing down of the sympathetic ("fight or flight") chemical outflow from the nervous system and in general producing a calm state in the nervous system.

There appears to be a peak onset of chemical action at 3 to 5 hours with negative effect of lowered blood pressure seem-ing to occur within 30 to 60 minutes of taking the medication.

The maximum drop in blood pressure seems to occur within 2 to 4 hours after medication.

While children seem to be less susceptible to this blood pressure drop, in adults it can sometimes be the limiting factor for the use of Catapres. The negative aspects and side effects of this medication include dry mouth, dizziness, some sedation, and lowered blood pressure. These seem to be fairly well tolerated and seem to attenuate over a series of days to weeks.

> *J. P. is a forty-two-year-old executive. Initially, he self-diagnosed his ADD after his son was diagnosed. Because his son has sleep difficulties as well as ADD, the boy was placed on clonidine and did very well.*
>
> *J. P. decided to "try out" his son's medication to see if it would have the same positive effect on him. Unfortunately, rather than slowly increasing the dosage, he took a full dose and promptly proceeded to feel lightheaded and dizzy and he ultimately passed out. He was taken to the emergency room, treated with fluids through the vein, as well as with medicines to counter the effects of the clonidine and he was ultimately referred to our office.*
>
> *He* did *make the correct diagnosis of ADD. But after a review of his history and physical exam, it turned out that J. P. was a runner with a slow pulse and low blood pressure, therefore clonidine was a* bad *choice for him. He was switched to Ritalin and is* doing well.

While Catapres is available as .1, .2, and .3 mg tablets, it is also available as a very effective clonidine patch that allows application of the medication once every week. The patch seems to be effective for 5 to 7 days, particularly in its role in blood pressure regulation.

While this seems silly to point out, caution has to be taken in using this patch, particularly in removing the old patch prior to placement of a new patch. We have had some serious complications in patients who thought the patch had fallen off, when it had only slid out of view, and they applied a second patch. This did, indeed, lead to serious lower blood pressure which, fortunately, was corrected with fluids and standard medical care. Nevertheless, we strongly advise caution with the clonidine patch.

Nontraditional Use of Anticonvulsants

Under this category of medications, one can list the more traditional anticonvulsants such as *Depakote* (valproic acid), *Dilantin* (diphenylhydantoin), and *Tegretol* (carbamazepine). All these medications have had their positive role in modifying moods, attention, thought, and behavior.

Tegretol specifically has become quite popular among psychiatrists in the use and control of manic depressive (or "bipolar") disorders. It has also had a great deal of positive benefit for depression. These medications have been around for a long time and are most traditionally used as standard anticonvulsant therapies.

A recent article described the role of Depakote and its positive impact on attention and learning in a young child who had an abnormal EEG but had no clinical seizures. With the Depakote medication there was profound improvement in this individual's thinking, as evidenced by a marked change in his handwriting while on the medication as compared to off. We have a great deal of experience with this medicine in patients with seizure disorders and it has recently been noted to have a positive effect in reducing the frequency and intensity of migraine headaches.

The literature has not expanded broadly into these medications and roles for attention disorders, yet we have had anecdotal involvement with these medications with positive effects. In addition, as neurologists we are quite comfortable with these medications and know the side effect profile quite well.

However, we would like to point to newer medications in this class of anticonvulsants. The first is *Neurontin* (gabapentin). This medication comes as capsules of 100, 300, and 400 mg. The exact mechanism of its action is unknown, even with regard to its antiseizure effect. It is chemically similar to GABA, which is a chemical messenger of the brain. GABA functions in an unknown capacity similar to other brain chemicals like serotonin, norepinephrin, and dopamine.

The recommended dose of this medication ranges from 300 to 600 mg three times per day, yet even for seizure management this dosage is somewhat variable. There were standard adverse side effects, as noted with other antiseizure medicines, quite similar to many of the other chemicals we listed earlier in this chapter, that affect the central nervous system. These include somnolence, dizziness, unsteadiness and imbalance, fatigue, and occasionally a sense of nervousness or restlessness.

With other anticonvulsant medications, such as Dilantin, Tegretol, and even Depakote, laboratory monitoring is needed. This is not so with Neurontin, and there is no requirement for blood testing, laboratory evaluation or monitoring of serum levels of kidney or liver function.

Of course, a standard medical evaluation is appropriate, particularly if there are side effects, yet this is certainly not a mandatory aspect of this medication. There is yet no definite conclusion in terms of the ultimate value of this medication for attention deficit disorder, yet, like some of the other anticonvulsant medications, the positive anecdotal response thus far warrants further studies.

Lamictal (lamotrigine) Here again, the chemical mechanism of activity of this medication is uncertain. It does not appear to inhibit or block the uptake of norepinephrine, dopamine, serotonin, or other centrally acting chemicals. The medication comes in tablets of 25, 100, 150, and 200 mg.

While this medication has been proven to be a very effective antiseizure medication—and indeed its indications include adjunct therapy in the treatment of partial seizures in adults with epilepsy—here again we have found positive anecdotal response to our patients being treated with this medication for attention deficit disorder.

Side effects have included unsteadiness, visual blurring, double vision, dizziness, nausea, and vomiting, as well as a sense of restlessness, muscle pains, and some confusion and difficulty with concentration.

The dosage of Lamictal, at least initially, is 50 mg once a day for two weeks, to be slowly and steadily titrated up to therapeutic benefit. We have attempted to monitor the dosage increase with the side effects, trying to minimize the medication's negative impact.

As with the medication Neurontin, it is unclear what long-term role this centrally acting chemical will have and what will be its ultimate value in attention deficit disorder.

Serotonin/Norepinephrine Reuptake Inhibitor

Effexor (venlafaxine HCL) We are very excited about Effexor. We feel that we may be at the dawn of a new era, on the threshold of discovering just how powerful this medication can be. We think that Effexor forms a second foundation in the chemical therapy for individuals with attention deficit disorder. While certainly Ritalin is a direct central nervous system stimulant, and has a very positive role in our patients, the fact that it is a controlled substance does mean that it also carries a risk of abuse potential. As a result, many physicians and patients alike are reluctant to proceed with Ritalin. We have had very positive response in our patient trials with Effexor, not only for depression, mood, and motivation, but also in attention disorders; some ADD patients have shown dramatic improvements.

Effexor is chemically different from any prior tricyclic, tetracyclic, or other antidepressant medication. Its mechanism of action seems to be that it is a potent inhibitor of serotonin and norepinephrine reuptake, as well as a weak inhibitor of dopamine reuptake.

This means that with fewer chemicals taken up by the brain tissue, there are more circulating chemical transmitters, thereby allowing the brain filter to stabilize itself for longer periods of time. This therefore allows for a more stable "chemical milieu," allowing for fewer disruptions of thought and attention, and greater control on mood, impulsivity, and behavior.

The medication comes in various dosages including tablets of 25, 37.5, 50, 75, and 100 mg. The recommended dose of Effexor is 75 mg per day, but we generally start our patients off at half of this dose and, based on age, sometimes one quarter of this dose. While the maximum dose can be titrated up to 225 mg per day, we have had very good results at 75 mg twice per day and have not found the need to increase the medication.

Although various side effects have been listed with Effexor, we have been pleased with the paucity of side effects experienced by our patients. General side effects include at times a sensation of restlessness, some sweating, mild stomach upset, and occasional constipation. In the first few days, there is a complaint of dry mouth and some fatigue and sleepiness, and some individuals have complained of difficulty with ejaculation or orgasm. Despite these mild side effects—which are quite a bit less severe and less disabling than some of the other medications mentioned—the positive effects have been dramatic.

We have had patients who have tried and failed numerous medications, but for whom this specific serotonin/norepinephrine reuptake inhibitor medication seems to be very effective in treating the depression, energy, fatigue, and motivation aspects often associated with ADD. In addition, Effexor's stimulation of the dopamine system seems to be effective for the direct attention improvements mentioned above.

There have been numerous trials performed on many of the centrally acting medications. The results of a number of recent trials performed on Effexor, as well as our personal experience, make this medication extremely promising as a formidable agent in the arsenal for therapy for individuals with attention deficit disorder.

New on the Horizon

New medications are coming out every month, although many of them will be available in Europe and Canada prior to approval by the Food and Drug Administration (FDA) for use in the United States. In addition to multiple new delivery systems—transdermal (through the skin), by nasal spray, by injection—that various companies are working on, there are also new combinations of medications.

One of the more exciting medications we are monitoring is modafinil, being marketed under the trade name *Provigil.* This medication seems to work on the adrenergic receptors of the brain, producing increased vigilance and increased alertness. The pharmaceutical company is currently seeking FDA approval for its use in treating *narcolepsy,* a severe sleep disorder. Multiple studies are available to document its efficacy in producing increases of stimulation and vigilance and subsequently improving the narcolepsy.

One particular study actually looked at the effect of Provigil on mood, fatigue, cognitive performance, and body temperature, revealing modafinil to be a good alternative to amphetamines for reducing the debilitating mood and cognitive defects of sleep deprivation or sleep loss. There also appeared to be a slightly decreased abuse potential of modafinil as compared to standard amphetamine/stimulant therapy.

While certainly this medication will have a dramatic impact in the treatment of narcolepsy and sleep disorders, a desirable carryover effect would be its role in attention, stimulating alertness, energy, and drive.

At the time of this printing, modafinil is not yet available for the general population, and Phase 4 trials under the direction of Cephalon are underway with the hopes that this medication may be available soon. ("Phase 4" is the final phase in drug research before approval by the FDA, which means that this medication has passed trials 1, 2, and 3, showing it to be safe and effective.)

Combining Medications

Each of the medications we've discussed have their various roles in the treatment of individuals with ADD. However, it is important to understand that sometimes more than one medication is necessary. Specifically, one medication may treat part of the problem (a central nervous system stimulant may affect energy, attention, and drive), but it may completely avoid intervention for additional problems, such as depression or fatigue.

It is absolutely appropriate in many cases to use a combination of therapies. First, a combination approach may deal most effectively with the wide variety of symptoms that individuals with ADD suffer. Next, it is often true that medications will have side effects and the side effects can be very well balanced with a second medication, thus allowing individuals to take a higher and more effective dose of the first medication. This is an important concept, as often the side effects are the limiting factor in using medications, before they can gain the full therapeutic benefit.

In addition, every individual with ADD is unique in his or her own way. For this reason, tailoring a treatment regimen is absolutely necessary, and, while some individuals respond well to central nervous system stimulants, others are better treated with serotonin or norepinephrine reuptake inhibitors. Still others may respond best to the nontraditional medications.

We think it is very important to keep an open mind in the management of ADD, particularly when it comes to using some of the more controlled substances. We do urge caution in the use of co-pharmacy (some individuals would call it *poly*-pharmacy, using many drugs to treat a specific disorder); specifically, we rarely introduce more than one new medicine at a time; otherwise, we would not know which medication produced which positive or negative effects.

Conclusion

As we have pointed out in this chapter, there are multiple options in the therapeutic regimen for treatment of adults with attention deficit disorder. While most people in the popular press have focused on Ritalin, there are also other options.

Our primary recommendation to readers is to proceed cautiously with medication trials, only under the supervision and guidance of a physician. Many of our adult patients come to us as they have been identified when they take their children in for diagnosis and evaluation. Using your child's medication may not be an appropriate form of therapy, and we urge our patients to use a great deal of caution in the initiation of therapy. Just as someone who suspects he has diabetes mellitus would not go out and initiate unsupervised use of insulin, we feel that individuals who suspect they may have a component of attention deficit disorder should not go out and use someone else's medications, or even try to self-medicate with over-the-counter remedies, until a diagnosis is firmly established. In addition, other significant neurologic illnesses should first be excluded, and a comprehensive and complete treatment plan outlined.

As we pointed out earlier, a diagnosis of attention deficit disorder is an *explanation,* not an excuse for behavior dysfunction. In addition, professionally diagnosed attention deficit disorder should be considered a lifelong illness and the goal of therapy should be complete control of this disorder. While ADD can never be "removed, cut out, or eliminated," it can be very well controlled and, with a comprehensive diagnostic and therapeutic approach, most patients should be able to live a relatively uninhibited and unencumbered life.

7

Other Treatments
for Adult ADD

━━━◦ᗰᒪ§ᒪᗰᙍ━━━

We frequently see patients who refuse to consider taking medications for their ADD. They often cite a fear of side effects or interactions with medications they are already taking, such as antidepressants, antihypertensives, or others. Other patients aren't clearly able to identify the reasons why they don't wish to take medications, but they refuse nonetheless.

Some patients fear taking medications such as Ritalin or other stimulants because of a family or personal history of drug abuse, and even when there is a very small risk of addiction or abuse, these patients still adamantly refuse to consider a short course of drug therapy.

It is true that there are some valid medical reasons for avoiding certain medications, particularly among the elderly. Patients with severe coronary disease or uncontrolled hypertension would not be good candidates for Ritalin therapy. And patients with irregular heartbeats should not take some of the tricyclic medications. Another factor is that concomitant use of alcohol could complicate virtually any of the drug regimens used in ADD. Although we feel that at least a trial of some of the commonly used medications for adult ADD might be worthwhile, we certainly respect a patient's wishes and will attempt to provide other treatment options.

In this chapter we will discuss various types of therapy that can compliment or, in some cases, replace medication therapy for adult attention deficit disorder. This chapter focuses on a variety of treatments, including psychotherapy and biofeedback, both effective options in dealing with the problems of attention deficit disorder.

Psychotherapy

One of us vividly recalls an experience during a psychiatry rotation in medical school. A closet Freudian at that time, he had some resistance to medication therapy and instead had great faith in the mental health powers of psychotherapy. On the first day of the clinical rotation, this eager medical student informed the professor of psychiatry that drugs were overused in psychiatry and that "delving into the problem" was more appropriate for psychiatric patients, including schizophrenics.

After listening patiently, the professor pointed out the behavior of some of the patients on the psychiatric floor. Some were bound in leather restraints, while others roamed aimlessly about the ward, often actively hallucinating. The professor had made his point quite clearly. If a psychotherapeutic intervention is to be successful, the patient has to be receptive, able to pay attention, and relatively in control of intrusive thoughts and emotions. Otherwise, he or she is unable to benefit from any type of psychotherapy.

While these psychotic patients were very sick and not as functional as most people with adult attention deficit disorder, the same considerations apply. It's unlikely that psychotherapy will be effective in a patient who has racing thoughts, gives in to frequent impulses, and has great difficulty sitting or lying down during the sessions. In these cases, certainly medication therapy is essential.

Why Psychotherapy?

Most of us have encountered foreigners who have learned English from nonnative speakers (other foreign people) or tapes or records. While these individuals may have large vocabularies and a fairly good understanding of the spoken language, they often commit various errors when attempting to speak our language. They haven't yet had the opportunity to converse regularly with native speakers who would provide them with the necessary feedback for developing a more functional command of English. As a result, they will continue to make the same errors over and over until they do converse with people whose native tongue is English.

Similarly, while the adult ADD patient may have some good response to medication and self-help books and other forms of education, she is likely to continue to commit the same errors and observe the same self-defeating and inappropriate patterns of behavior unless she obtains adequate feedback from a "native speaker"—in this case, a psychotherapist. In the course of psychotherapy the patient will have the opportunity to receive professional feedback on the myriad issues facing an adult with ADD.

How Patients React to Their ADD Diagnosis

One of the first issues that arises in any psychotherapeutic treatment program is the patient's reaction to diagnosis. Many patients are relieved to find that their problems are not a result of being "bad" or having some moral weakness. Others may be bitter and feel a sense of hopelessness about the diagnosis and its implications for the future.

Some individuals react with a deep sense of anger when the diagnosis is determined. They're unreasonably angry with themselves that they have the disease in the first place. They are also often angry with many individuals in their past who have ignorantly "assumed the worst" about them when confronted with their forgetfulness, difficulty paying attention, impulsiveness, and inappropriate behavior.

At this point, the therapist should actively promote a sense of optimism in the patient, who needs to understand that while she does have a chronic neurologic disease with far-reaching consequences, there is hope for the future. The person with ADD must develop confidence that self-defeating behavior patterns are not ironclad DNA labyrinths in which they are hopelessly entrapped for eternity. She also must learn to forgive the past and be convinced that the failure-directed impulses that have led them to disaster in the past can be disarmed.

Therapists Should Promote Self-Education

The therapist cannot be with the patient twenty-four hours a day, so the patient must learn from various sources about the illness, in particular by reading books, attending lectures, and going to support group meetings for adults with ADD. Usually the therapist will be a major source of education about the disease. During therapy the patient will have opportunities to discuss the various sources of frustration with the therapist. Occasionally, the therapist will assume a directing role using his past experience with ADD to seek out the issues that more commonly affect those suffering from this illness. Informing the patient how this diagnosis often affects families and work is invaluable to the patient.

Teaching the Person with ADD How to Change

Often, the person with ADD will have very little insight into the various patterns that lead to failure. He may be unable to identify the social ineptness that is patently obvious to everyone around him.

Social interaction can be compared to a soccer match that involves a very complex set of rules involving more than some individuals kicking a ball about a field. A spectator cannot walk down from the stands and begin kicking the ball around—that is against the rules. It's also important for team players to have a keen sense of what is going on at all times—where the goal is, and the position of opponents and teammates.

The adult ADDer may have spent a lifetime of walking into complex situations like our soccer game, yet he was completely unaware of errors that others could see immediately. For example, the importance of eye contact, displaying an interest in others, and exchanging social pleasantries are recognized by most people. But the ADDer may have never quite comprehended their importance in everyday social life. And the adult world is a very unforgiving place for individuals who do not follow the rules.

An adult with ADD often also has problems at home that are directly related to the attention deficit disorder. The forgetfulness, impulsiveness, and apparent insensitivities of many people with ADD can all lead to great disharmony in the family setting.

Edward T. was a successful businessman who had known for years that he had attention deficit disorder; consequently, he was terribly concerned that his children would also have the illness; he saw that possibility as a very serious problem.

So every day, when Edward came home from work, he would immediately start an intense interrogation of his children. What had they done during the day, and what did they expect to accomplish during the evening? As a result of this unpleasant questioning, Edward's children began to seek any number of excuses to avoid being "grilled."

Through counseling, Edward was able to realize that it was possible to demonstrate concern and be a

good parent without actually questioning the children in
a negative way. As a result, the parent-child relationship
was greatly improved for Edward and his family.

Self-esteem issues can be quite disabling for a person
with ADD. An expectation of failure can prevent him from
ever being successful and can also destroy his ability to recognize and appreciate genuine successes. The effective therapist reassures the patient that he is not unique in having this
approach to life, and that this fear of failure can be changed,
although a large degree of effort will be required.

It is okay for the therapist to say many positive things
to the adult ADDer on a frequent basis and to encourage
other family members to do so. Care must be devoted also at
this point to establish a recognition in the patient that attention deficit disorder is an *explanation* of his behavior, and not
an excuse.

Problems surrounding activity continuity, i.e. the ability to
sustain meaningful participation in a given task or effort, can
be particularly disabling for individuals suffering from this
disease. ADDers can be totally absorbed with a particular
emotion or activity one minute but may have totally forgotten
it a minute later. This feature of ADD makes learning from
mistakes very difficult for ADDers. The therapist can help the
patient maintain the continuity that is necessary to avoid
making the same mistake repeatedly by pointing out errors to
her. It is particularly in this area that the therapist's knowledge about and commitment to the patient are of greatest
importance.

The therapist should know about the projects in which
the ADDer is involved and should follow these in a goal-
directed manner, providing criticism or direction or praise
appropriately. The therapist should also remind the patient of
similar experiences in the past and empower the patient with
strategies to break out of the ADDer's seemingly limitless
ability to "achieve failure" with increasing efficiency.

The therapist will also involve other issues related to adults with ADD, including recognition of other illnesses that may complicate the picture, such as alcohol or drug abuse, or depression. Individuals with attention deficit disorder may have been abused in the past. Issues related to abuse may also need specific focus during the psychotherapy.

Often other family members are drawn into the psychotherapeutic regimen, and sometimes they may be able assume some of the functions of the therapist. (See chapter 1 for more information on how ADD affects one's family and friends.)

Group Therapy and ADD Support Groups

Group therapy is often an especially effective form of therapy in adult attention deficit disorder because one of the most commonly described emotions in individuals with ADD is the sense of being different. Many people with ADD are totally convinced that they are unlike anyone else and more or less a freak of nature. Being in the room with other individuals with similar problems can have a very dramatic and immediate effect on someone suffering from this disorder. Psychiatrist Edward Hallowell describes this as a sense of "connectiveness." It can be a great source of relief to hear that others in one's community have had similar problems and face similar difficulties with regard to work, family life, etc. Individuals can vent not only their successes but also teach the coping strategies they have personally developed to others. Individuals in the session groups can learn from the other members and thus not have to "reinvent the wheel."

Many people also find that attending ADD support groups is another successful adjunct to individual or group therapy, either instead of or in addition to group therapy.

We feel that psychotherapy is an absolutely necessary feature of any effective strategy for attention deficit disorder at any age. We realize that many adult ADD sufferers may have had bad experiences in the past with psychotherapy, but suggest that this has been because of incorrect or incomplete diagnosis. The therapy will provide a focus for education, insight, and resolution of residual resentment; will educate the patient about the condition itself and will help her step off the "treadmill of frustration" and end the cycle of self-defeating attitudes and patterns of behavior.

Cognitive-Behavioral Therapy

There are different forms of therapy, but the kind that is probably most effective for people with ADD is *cognitive-behavioral therapy*. It is typically performed on a one-to-one basis between the patient and therapist. The program is directed toward specific problems that a patient may be having, such as problems with self-esteem, organization, and social interaction.

Cognitive-behavioral therapy helps to promote self-regulation of the patient's behavior. It also teaches the person how to use an internal dialogue in which he can become his own "coach" and direct his behaviors more efficiently. The efficacy of cognitive therapy has been studied more in children than adults, thus very little data supports its use in adults with attention deficit disorder.

Biofeedback

Biofeedback is a fascinating technology that has been used for various medical problems such as headaches, (including migraine), high blood pressure, stress management and, more recently, attention deficit disorder. For the purpose of our discussion, the type of biofeedback we will discuss is based on influencing the brain wave pattern or electroencephalogram (EEG). The strategy is based on teaching the subject to control physiologic processes, which normally occur on an involuntary basis. This therapy does not involve any pain and is entirely noninvasive. Electrodes are placed on the scalp as well as in both ears.

The activity of the brain is amplified electronically and the various brain wave patterns are connected to some type of visual display such as a video game. The different types of brain wave patterns will affect the video game in different ways. By repeated trials, the patient learns to control the video game and, at the same time, the brain wave activity.

This type of therapy has been studied more in children than in adults. Up to eighty visits, costing up to $100 each, may be needed. As Dr. Russell Barkley suggests in his book, *Taking Charge of ADHD*, the money spent on this type of therapy would pay for a very large amount of traditional psychotherapy as well as stimulant medication.

Sessions last approximately 40 minutes and are performed from one to five times weekly. As a general rule, some improvement is noted within the first ten visits. Studies have suggested that the improvement is permanent. While this therapy cannot be regarded as "mainstream" at this point, the preliminary indicators are that this will be a powerful technique in the treatment of attention deficit disorder.

More widespread use of this therapy and possible future technological advances may make biofeedback a much more economically viable tool in the treatment of attention deficit disorder. Unquestionably, much more will be written on this subject in the future.

Other Therapies for ADD

There are other therapies that have been tried for people with ADD, including both special training, non-prescription drugs, and techniques. We will cover the primary ones in this section, and tell you whether we think they work or not.

Auditory Integration Therapy (AIT) *Auditory integration therapy* uses sensory integration and is based on the premise that the key problem in people with ADD is that the central nervous system is working as an inefficient filter. With this therapy, various sound frequencies are presented using standard equipment and technology, and the goal is to increase sensory awareness. Music is played at various speeds and patterns with various frequencies, using a blocking approach.

Auditory integration therapy is most frequently used for individuals with autism, but has also been used experimentally with some individuals with ADD. (Many are children.) After ten days of thirty- to sixty-minute sessions twice per day, you can often see a dramatic improvement in a person's sound discrimination.

If the auditory process is deficient in its functioning—which may explain the easy distractibility seen in ADD—then resetting the "auditory system" by having it process and filter a complete spectrum of frequencies may be appropriate.

The jury is certainly still out on this therapy, however, so it is not yet considered an approved therapy for individuals with ADD. However, as a personal experience, this has been performed on Dr. Kandel's child, with rather positive results. It appears that the only negative to this treatment is the cost, and thus it certainly may be worthwhile (as long as it does not displace other more traditional and more effective therapies).

Dietary Intervention

Dietary control and the impact of nutrition have both been hot topics over the past decade. Previously, salicylates were considered to be irritants to the nervous system, as well as sugar, artificial food colorings and flavorings, among a number of other food "no-nos." Yet most research has failed to support the value of dietary intervention as positive for individuals with ADD.

We do not maintain any specific "ADD diet." However, obtaining good general health is certainly reasonable in any medical illness, and therefore we recommend that our patients maintain a well-balanced diet, with low cholesterol, low fat, and high in the complement of complete food groups. As in anything else, common sense and health care go a long way.

Megavitamins and Mineral Supplements

Many articles have been written about a variety of vitamin therapies and their possible impact on ADD. Virtually every company on the market has their own name brand of vigilance-enhancing vitamins or nutrition supplements. We cannot say with certainty whether any of these has a positive effect, although some may, indeed, carry a positive *placebo* effect. (You *think* you feel better because you think the medicine is supposed to work. Therefore, you do feel better, even if it's a sugar pill you took. The placebo effect is a positive self-fulfilling prophecy.)

We recommend antioxidant vitamins such as vitamin E and vitamin C (800 IU and 1000 mg respectively), as well as a B complex vitamin. A multivitamin with magnesium is certainly very appropriate for good general health and nutrition. Much of this can be offset if the patient would follow and maintain a well-balanced diet. Yet eating right is often difficult if not impossible with individuals with ADD who either eat on the run, are forgetful, or simply eat whatever is at hand.

Because excessive vitamin intake can cause problems (e.g., too much vitamin A can lead to liver involvement, while too much vitamin C can lead to kidney stones), moderation is important when it comes to a megavitamin, multivitamin, and mineral supplements. Follow the directions on the label and don't take too many pills. If one would be good, this doesn't mean that three or more would be better—this is not good reasoning at all.

The Yeast of Your Problems

Many popular holistic books are available on the subject of yeast and its relation to health. Some authors who practice

Eastern or nontraditional medicine implicate a Candida (yeast) as the culprit for all medical ills. Candida is present in the body of every human, although it is usually kept in check by a positive immune system and by the normal bacteria that exists in all of us.

It is true that when the immune system is weakened or is overactive in an inappropriate way, Candida can overgrow. In women this is often seen following antibiotic use as a vaginal yeast infection. This problem can also occur anywhere in the alimentary (food) tract from the mouth through the food tube to the stomach or intestines.

While yeast has been implicated in a multitude of medical disorders, at present there is no clear or compelling evidence that it plays any significant role in ADD. As a result, we don't recommend yeast avoidance or yeast suppression as a therapy for individuals with ADD.

Kinesiology

Chiropractic care, manipulation care, and hands-on healing all have a role in our society today, and we frequently work with chiropractic physicians when it comes to managing patients with soft tissue injuries and musculoskeletal disorders.

One problem, however, is that some chiropractors (a minority of them) state that they can cure *any* medical illness by simple spinal manipulation. They feel that the skeletal alignment has control over every bodily function; consequently, they believe an alignment problem can cause significant dysfunction, including inability to "gaze shift," that is, to focus the eyes when turning the head. Therapy includes recurrent spinal manipulation and adjustments, proper body mechanics, and proper body posture.

We believe that chiropractic care has a strong place in preventive care and wellness, but we are not at all convinced that it has a strong place in treating individuals with ADD.

Eye Muscle Training

Eye muscle training was popular in past years and, though it has since fallen out of favor, there are still a number of individuals who continue to believe strongly that the fundamental difficulty with individuals with ADD is poor visual processing, due to poor functioning of the eye muscles. They believe that if the eyes do not focus symmetrically on an object, then the brain must certainly be receiving two objects, confusing the brain and causing the distraction.

More recent evidence has pointed out that most cognitive reading and language disorders are not so much a problem of receiving the sensory input (seeing the object), but rather a problem in the central nervous system, the thinking part of the brain, and also the part that does the processing. In other words, the computer of the brain is not functioning at an appropriate level, and no degree of retraining eye muscles will correct this problem. We urge our patients not to settle for eye muscle training to treat their ADD.

Additional Pharmacological Therapies

Many people, including reporters in the popular press, have for some time been very intrigued by nontraditional medication therapies. As of this writing, the most popular substance being touted for ADD is *pycnogenol.* Some people believe that because it is "natural," it must also be safe, as well as hopefully effective. (We might remind them that there are many deadly poisons in nature. Pycnogenol is not poisonous, but you should never take an excessive amount of this substance.)

Some people have reported that after they've started taking pycnogenol, they immediately began functioning at a higher level, with workload and school performance dramatically improving. We have not actually seen this happen, and feel strongly that this should be viewed with careful optimism.

Pycnogenol, a derivative of the pine tree, is an antioxidant, and has minimal side effects when taken in moderate amounts. We are not adverse to our patients trying pyc-nogenol, as some individuals will use 50 mg capsules twice per day. We are always interested in individual reports, and if you are on pycnogenol or if you find that this medication has produced any specific negative or positive effects, we would like to hear about this. Please see page 250 for our 800 phone number, as well as our address.

Nontraditional Medicines

We would be remiss if we left out the nontraditional medications that are best considered holistic. The following is a brief overview of "nontraditional" medicines, as well as their roles and presumed usages:

Gingko This has been touted as an energy pill, longevity pill, as well as a "smart drug." It comes in many forms, can be purchased over the counter, certainly at the health food stores, and is widely available. In some individuals we have seen who have used this medication, there have been no apparent negative side effects, and some people have claimed increased energy and attention.

Ginseng While this is originally a Chinese chemical, coming from a root, it seems to have some impact on the central nervous system, as well as the cardiovascular system. Some individuals seem to feel that this helps with the serum glucose levels (diabetes), as well as with the immune system and thought inattention. It may have some positive impact on neurotransmitter release and reuptake, very much like some of the prescription antidepressants. This, however, is not entirely clear.

Garlic This herb has a longstanding history of medicinal use. It seems to have some positive effect for antibacterial and antiviral properties, and seems to reduce atherosclerotic vascular disease. It is uncertain if this actually does improve thought or attention, as claimed.

Green tea   This is a widely cultivated herb, very popular throughout the world, seeming to have a positive impact on energy and stamina. It is considered an "antioxidant" with multiple organ systems gaining benefit from its use. It is not clear whether the central nervous system, thought process, and inattention are improved with this.

Echinaceae   This naturally occurring substance is reported to stimulate the immune system. It seems to reduce allergic reactions and reduce fever following infections.

Valerian   This herb is considered to be a natural relaxant, very much akin to the prescription Valium. It is considered safe, nonhabitforming, and seems to be very effective for sleep initiation. As we do see this as a significant problem in our patients with ADD, this sometimes improves sleep initiation and maintenance, reduces early morning awakening, and leaves a generalized calm state. Valerian comes in many different forms and, although it is not standardized, a trial and error usage seems to be most effective.

Choline   Many nutritionists feel that this is a chemical best characterized as within the B complex family. No clear routine allowance or daily minimum has been set, yet we do feel that this agent seems to be very important for the nervous system. Previously, this was considered to be a cornerstone of Alzheimer disease and we do feel that choline is very necessary for the positive and normal functioning of the nerve cells throughout the brain. Movement disorders, Parkinson's disease, and cognitive dysfunction have all been linked to choline deficiency. This chemical seems to have a strong feedback mechanism, providing release of neurotransmitters, chemical messengers of the brain, and these seem to affect mood, memory, and learning.

Calcium/magnesium   These are two minerals and these work as copilots in helping vitamins achieve their maximum function. Indeed, as we discussed, when dealing with patients with migraine disorders it is very clear that B complex alone, or B_{12} alone, will not be as effective as B complex combined with magnesium. It seems the magnesium is very important in helping the B complex get where it needs to go. One may simply think of this as a taxi, with the B complex being the passenger and the magnesium and calcium being the driver.

Melatonin Melatonin is a naturally occurring hormone existing in all of us, produced by the pineal gland, a small structure at the center of the brain. This seems to be very important in setting rhythms, the day and night cycle, and is particularly important in setting seasonal variations in our bodies' rhythms. We might compare the action of this substance to the red-breasted robin knowing when to mate, and when to be dormant. The pineal gland secretes this melatonin and lets us "know" when to be active and when to be at rest.

Deficiencies in melatonin are linked with muscular aches and pains, mood disorders, lassitude, and fatigue. In addition, decreased attention and concentration have been noted in individuals with melatonin deficiencies. We have had a number of success stories with our patients using melatonin, particularly using it as a sleep medication. This is discussed more completely in numerous popular journals, as well as in our books *Migraine—What Works!* and *Back Pain—What Works!*

Essential Fatty Acids In this era of high cholesterol, high triglycerides, fatty blood and atherosclerosis, many people have come to believe that all fats are bad and should be eradicated completely. This certainly is not true at all. There are two essential fatty acids—eicosapentaenoic acid (EPA), and docosahexaenoic acid (DHA)—that seem to actually strengthen various cellular organisms within our body, improve our immune system, reduce fatty blood and, most importantly, seem to serve a protective mechanism for the nervous system.

Some believe that fatty acids are also important in the healing for multiple sclerosis attacks. While these fatty acids are routinely derived from cold water fish oil, they can also be found in some plants. Some people would refer to these as "primrose oil." Although we think there may be a valid role in general nutrition for these oils, we recommend caution; as with any other body fats and oils, they may reduce absorption of other chemicals, nutrients, and vitamins.

These nontraditional, nonprescription chemicals are meant to be an incomplete reference to the numerous therapies available for individuals with ADD. While we profess to be traditional neurologists, practicing mainstream neurology, we are aware of our patients' longing to find a cure by whatever means. Many of our patients have already experimented with one or more of these therapies.

A word of caution: People with ADD often have a tendency to leap before they look, and impulsivity, a hallmark of ADD, can get some of our patients in trouble. For example, using allergy medicines that have been touted as effective for ADD may be fine in certain individuals. But if there is any degree of heart disease, lung disease, or other medical process, such medication could be disastrous. Also, what works for one individual may be entirely wrong for another. We cannot stress too strongly that you should *be extremely cautious in using some of the nonprescribed medications.*

We recommend that you discuss this thoroughly with your treating physician, particularly if you are very interested in pursuing one or more of these therapeutic options. If your physician has experience with individuals with ADD, then she can intelligently explain the pros and cons in your individual case and can tailor a specific, personalized treatment regimen that is exactly right for you.

8

Coping with ADD:
Self-Help Strategies
for Daily Problems

———⟨⟨⟨⟨⟨ ⟩ ⟩⟩⟩⟩———

A broad array of life issues—including physical, emotional, financial, and social issues—are directly affected by attention deficit disorder. In this chapter, we'll cover major health issues that you may experience in addition to ADD and that are often *caused* by ADD—issues such as serious sleep disorders and problems with driving.

We will also discuss two very important aspects of the patient with attention deficit disorder: financial and social issues. Each can affect an individual's everyday life in profound ways.

Wellness, Illness, or None of the Above?

Most of our patients with attention deficit disorder come to us with complaints of disorganized thought, confusion, decreased concentration, and occasionally decreased energy or stamina. Often our patients are secondarily diagnosed as having ADD when they appear with other, more traditional neurologic disorders such as neck pain, back pain, migraine, or carpal tunnel syndrome.

One common denominator we've noticed among our ADD patients is that most of them simply don't take the time to pay attention to their general health. On the one hand, many of our patients with ADD describe their condition as a blessing as well as a curse. They feel they gain a great deal of inspiration, insight, and sometimes energy and creativity from their disorder.

Another common feature is that they often become hyperfocused, concentrating on one issue or problem to the exclusion of all else. Have you ever sat at your computer or desk for hours on end while working on a project, and forgotten to eat, to go to the bathroom, to take a break at all? Only at the end of the work project do you get up and suddenly notice that you have a stiff neck, full bladder, an empty, angry upset stomach. And you may well pay it for the next series of hours or days.

This is a classic scenario, but is only the tip of the iceberg. Patients with ADD also have a problem with distractibility and with impulse control. Consequently, these traits make sticking to a general fitness and medical schedule for wellness seemingly impossible.

> *Bill P., a successful forty-four-year-old, self-employed businessman, was instructed by us to start a general fitness exercise program for his lower back pain. Realizing Bill also had attention deficit disorder, we gave him a booklet for back exercises, and outlined numerous options for exercise regimen.*
>
> *But at the third follow-up visit for his failed back syndrome, it was painfully clear to both doctor and patient that Bill had absolutely forgotten all of the instructions given to him and had lost the booklet. He was supposed to join the fitness club for his exercise program. Here's what happened.*

*First, he actually did join the fitness club, and
decided he would work with the general fitness trainer,
doing a general warm-up program, mild aerobic session,
and a light weight-training session. All of this seemed
reasonable. But then Bill saw the Stairmaster, and
decided instead that he should do thirty to forty minutes
of Stairmaster activity a day. However, after a few days,
he changed his mind and concluded that the treadmill
would be a far more effective measure for aerobic activity
and tried thirty to forty minutes of treadmill exercise.*

*Bill started and then stopped his back exercises, his
stretching, and he often would forget to do his thorough
warm-up exercises for his back pain. Consequently, he
suffered from multiple, very painful flare-ups.*

*What did Bill conclude from this experience? That an
exercise program wouldn't work for his back pain syndrome. When Bill told us about his problems with maintaining the exercise we so urgently recommended, we
discussed some corrective action he could take. One plan
was to hire a personal trainer and follow the prescribed
plan on a workout sheet for three hours per week. (Leaving the workout sheet at the health club, where it would
not be lost!) This plan would allow him to arrive at the
workout center, do a brief warm-up, followed by thirty to
forty minutes of directed exercises for his lower back,
performed in a stepwise, sequential fashion.*

*We instructed Bill to chart each of these exercises
on his workout sheet and record them at each visit. He
was also instructed to fax the workout sheet to us on a
weekly basis, so it would ensure that someone was
looking over his shoulder.*

*This plan worked. After three months of this regi-
men, Bill had progressed, had actually increased his
workout activities to ninety minutes three times per
week, with a thirty-minute home exercise regimen once
to twice per week. At the end of this interval, Bill's back*

was better, and although he did continue to sit for too long a period of time, and did lift, bend, and twist in an inappropriate fashion on too many occasions, the exercises made it possible for him to continue his routine activities, and his back pain was markedly reduced.

The key aspect of this scenario is that it took multiple office visits, and only with a great deal of questioning was it revealed that Bill's easy distractibility and inability to stay on target were potent enemies in preventing him from recovering from his spine pain condition.

This is just one illustration of how ADD can affect general health, which goes back to the key aspect of making sure that you, as a person with ADD:

1. Understand the physician's orders for any medical illness.
2. Get those instructions in writing.
3. Have someone check to make sure those instructions are being followed.
4. Keep a simple diary of what is being done (or not being done) to follow the instructions.

Habit Substitution

Many patients with attention deficit disorder often have an associated addictive personality. We see a great number of individuals who have "co-morbid" issues of smoking or drinking alcohol too much. Even such behaviors as gambling to excess can be associated with attention deficit disorder. How do you deal with a bad habit that is impairing your health?

One of the fundamental techniques of behavior modification is habit substitution. If health professionals can substitute a healthy or positive behavior habit for one that is destructive, it is virtually impossible to continue the destructive habit. For example, if you believe that the excitement and danger of using illicit drugs is what draws the person with ADD, it might be a good idea to substitute a less negative but also exciting activity—such as skydiving.

If you incorporate an exercise regimen as a habit that becomes ultimately ingrained, it then becomes virtually impossible to continue smoking or drinking to excess. As anyone who works out or exercises on a frequent basis knows, it is very unpleasant (and unlikely) to work out in an aerobic fashion, with resistance training, and then reach for a cigarette or cigar. Likewise, someone who is very health conscious and physically fit would be unlikely to drink to excess, as the two behaviors and habits are contradictory.

General Inattention to Health

It is clear from our patients that there is a general inattention to their health rather than a directed neglect. They just don't think about it that much, if at all. For example, hyperfocusing on a certain activity can lead to a patients' skipping or missing one or two meals at a time, often causing them to grab for whatever is available. This could include attempting a fast-food fix rather than a well-balanced nutritional meal, which may take more time to prepare.

As discussed in chapter 2 on the causes of ADD, researchers originally believed that poor diet played a significant role—such as diets high in sugar, particularly in children with ADD. Now we realize this is probably not true. Nevertheless, there has been some concern over the body's craving for certain foods and items, particularly in chronic deficiency states. Such deficiencies may lead to inappropriate choices when it comes to general nutrition.

Of course, fast food is okay on an occasional basis, but we see people with ADD over-relying on fast food. It is important to plan time into your schedule to make that salad and vegetable or meat dish, rather than habitually ordering in a pizza. Budgeting time for planning and preparing a nutritious meal will pay off in your health. You'll save money, too. (Fast food can be very pricey.)

Your Sleep Cycle: Crash and Burn?

The sleep cycle is a very important issue for many people with ADD because so many experience problems, primarily insomnia. Often people with ADD can acquire what is known to sleep specialists as a "sleep debt." This means patients often rob their bodies of their necessary amounts of sleep on a twenty-four-hour-cycle basis, only to require a catch-up period later in the week or even later in the month. For example, you may be a hard-charging person all week, and then crumple up and want to sleep all weekend.

This constant shifting of sleep, which in many other aspects of life activities is referred to as "robbing Peter to pay Paul," ultimately takes it toll on the body. Sleep deprivation and sleep debt are both associated with mood change, mood swings, and irritability. They are also almost always associated with excessive daytime sleepiness, which can often be mistaken for laziness and inattention. In the work force, employees who are sleepy or apparently lazy during the day are regarded as underproductive—and dispensable.

Sleep disturbance also feeds into the distractibility syndrome, setting up a classic downward spiral; patients with ADD often are hyperfocused, do not listen to their biological clocks, stay up late finishing projects or working on creative new ideas, only to oversleep the next morning, be exhausted, fatigued, perform poorly, be tardy, be unable to complete tasks on a timely basis. This process eventually leads to a low self-esteem as patients constantly set themselves up for failure. *Remember, this is not intentional behavior, and is certainly not a planned self-destructive agenda.* But the result is the same as if you had planned it.

This sleep cycle problem also leads to inattentiveness during the day, which is a central part of the ADD syndrome. Sleep-cycle disruption may explain why some individuals are better in the morning than they are in the afternoon with regard to concentration. It's also true that particularly in the early afternoon we all have a natural tendency to want to "take a siesta." This is the time when our patients with ADD seem to fail miserably.

Until you resolve your sleep problem, try to avoid scheduling critically important meetings or decision making. The worst time for the person with ADD (a difficult time for most people) is right after lunch. As any public speaker knows, you don't want to speak directly after lunch. Whenever possible, plan a light schedule for at least an hour after lunch. And work to resolve that sleep problem!

We address sleep problems with a very regimented lifestyle plan. We explain to our patients that it is important that they maintain a twenty-four-hour cycle, with a sleep/wake state that is appropriate for their work and social activities. This should be maintained on a seven-day-per-week basis. It does no good to work hard to maintain your alertness and attention during the weekdays, only to fall apart on the weekends because of staying up too late or sleeping too late the next day.

We also urge avoidance of stimulants such as caffeine before bedtime. Caffeine or other stimulants often excite thoughts and ideas, making it virtually impossible for the ADDer to settle down. (Also, getting up two or three times a night to use the bathroom is no way to get into a deep, uninterrupted sleep pattern.)

We also recommend that our patients set time limits on their activities and use some low- or high-tech devices (see chapter 9 on technology fixes) to make sure they maintain their work, social, and play schedule in a reasonable fashion. This may be as simple as setting an egg timer when someone is sitting in front of a computer, to as complex as having a device that beeps. Or it could be as low-tech as having a spouse or loved one remind you, "Honey, you've been at that long enough; it's time to come to bed."

We cannot tell you how many disagreements have been aired in our examination rooms over the issue of time. "He never comes to bed." "She's always up doing projects." "I can't ever seem to have any time with him." (This issue is discussed further in chapter 11, on issues related to patients with ADD and their friends and family.)

Another suggestion is to avoid all alcoholic beverages before bedtime. You may think that "just a nightcap will help me fall asleep." It may initially make you drowsy, but the problem is that alcohol irritates, inflames, and depresses the central nervous system. As a result, within the next few hours there will be a rebound effect, and subsequently a stimulant effect on the brain. Consequently, this nightcap to get you to sleep can cause you to wake up in the middle of the night, and have trouble falling back to sleep. This is why individuals who have alcohol beverages in mid evening can often be drowsy throughout the night but later on are wide awake and ready to keep going.

Avoid catnaps during the day. Although brief naps can allow patients to recharge themselves for a short period of time, this practice almost certainly guarantees that they continue their deranged sleep cycle on a chronic basis.

Don't go to bed mad. One of the simplest suggestions we make to our patients is not to go to bed angry or stressed. Although this sounds quite simple, in reality it can be difficult, as many of our patients take their problems to bed. This virtually guarantees that your mind will be distracted by a number of events or issues from earlier in the day, or tomorrow. You will rehash these thoughts over and over, and consequently you will have a poor sleep cycle.

We've told you what *not* to do, and now we'll offer some suggestions on what you *should do* to fall asleep:

1. Work on, practice, and develop positive relaxation techniques to initiate drowsiness and restfulness.

2. Be assertive—prepare your sleep environment to make it comfortable for you. Specifically eliminate activity, noises, or sounds that keep you awake. Many individuals tell us that with "white noise" or soothing background noise, they can effectively block out irritating sounds and actually allow themselves not to concentrate on "a thousand and one other thoughts."

3. Check with your doctor and pharmacist for guidance. Frequently, even medications that have been taken for a long period of time, or medicines that your physician has told you won't have any side effects may in fact have a stimulant effect. It is important to check on this, as there is almost always more than one medication for any one illness (and, as we've said before, different people react differently to medications).

   Don't be afraid to tell your physician that this disruption in your sleep cycle is an "issue." It certainly is an issue when you suffer from the multiple consequences it can produce.

In addition to those general concepts for preparing for a proper sleep cycle, some more specific suggestions are often helpful. For example, *L-Tryptophan,* an amino acid has been noted to be quite helpful in getting to sleep. This product is readily available in most pharmacies, health food stores, and groceries. In addition, foods high in L-Tryptophan content include bananas, yogurt, dates, and milk. (See? Mom was right when she told you to drink a nice glass of warm milk before bed.)

In addition, certain vitamins and supplements have also been found somewhat helpful in patients' getting to sleep, such as vitamin B_3, as well as calcium and magnesium. Also helpful are such herbs as valerian root and passion flower.

Of course, there are also traditional sleep medications. We have had a great deal of success using the medication *Ambien* for sleep initiation and maintenance. It produces very little hangover effect the next morning. We are also very excited about some European research on the medication *Modafinil,* which seems to be very helpful for excessive daytime somnolence. Although Modafinil is not yet available in the United States, we feel that this and medications like it will hold great promise for some of our patients, not only with sleep initiation but also with alertness, attention, and energy for those days when the sleep cycle has been significantly deranged.

Don't Forget to Take Your Medicine

One problem many people with ADD face chronically is their inability to remember to take prescription medications for other medical problems, such as high blood pressure, sugar diabetes, or thyroid disease. Even without ADD, it is hard enough for patients to remember twice or three-times-a-day dosage regimens, but adding the extra burden of attention deficit disorder makes this task virtually impossible.

We know it's hard, but it's really necessary that you follow your physician's instructions with regard to medication usage, and also that you be very cautious and careful to take your medications on time and in the proper dosage. It is not adequate to remember to take a pill two or three hours late; this may have disastrous effects.

Susan B. is one of our patients who has ADD, but she also is followed by her general medical physician for high blood pressure. She has been on a central nervous system stimulant, as well as a beta blocker and had done quite well (see further discussion of medications and ADD in chapter 6). However, Susan forgot to take her high blood pressure medications for a day and a half. Upon remembering these, she took triple the amount to "catch up"—but she didn't contact her family physician's office first. She fainted, struck the back of her head, and caused a severe neck sprain—a mild laceration to the back of her scalp. Fortunately, this did not lead to any serious medical complications, other than the high cost of the emergency room visit and the embarrassment and frustration that she caused the problem herself.

Susan's experience is a classic example of under- or overdosing medication because of inability to keep track of a medication schedule.

In our next chapter, on technology devices, we discuss high and low-tech devices for making sure you can maintain your treatment regimen, even if it's as simple as having a watch that beeps, carrying around a pillbox, placing your medication physically on your computer keyboard or packing it with your lunch or placing it on the table for breakfast, lunch, or dinner.

Amy K. created a little ritual to remember to take her medication. "I'd stop for soda on the way to work, get back in the car, take the pills, and drive to work."

One man told us he uses a simple memory device. He puts his medication next to his toothbrush. "I picture a large prescription bottle on my head while I brush my teeth. Sounds crazy. But it works for me."

Frank R. says sometimes he forgets his medications, but he keeps some extras in his briefcase. "On those days when I forget whether I've taken my Ritalin, I just wait to see if the 'fog' lifts. If it does, I know I've taken it. If not, I take one of the extra pills in my briefcase."

Follow the Doctor's Orders

A lot of people with ADD have trouble complying with the physician's instructions, even beyond taking the medication. Although this may sound trivial, it's not. People with ADD certainly understand the issues of losing instructions, as well as the problem of being distracted. (Tell the truth, now: how often have you left a physician's office and remembered each and every item the physician discussed during the ten- or fifteen-minute office visit? If you're like any of our patients, if you get 50 percent of what was said, you're way ahead of the game.) This is also a problem in the workplace, where employees with ADD may seem to be listening intently, then they leave and do half or less of what they were instructed. (See chapter 12, on workplace issues.)

There are some very simple ways to remember the doctor's orders. First of all, take a notepad and pen with you when you see the doctor and jot down notes during the visit. Even if it's quite distracting to you and the physician, this practice can be helpful. Using a tape recorder to record the session and then playing it back and taking notes at home later on may be a reasonable course for you to follow. Asking the physician for a copy of his instructions prior to the end of the appointment may be a good idea, too. Often on the physician's bill there will be notations regarding the patient's illness, as well as any instructions for the staff to follow. These often have a handwritten outline of the instructions that the physician reviewed with you.

Lastly, take the physician's business card, or ask for a contact person in the physician's office. Asking the nurse to go over any further instructions can actually be a life-saver in terms of making sure that each and every item the physician discussed is being conveyed to you.

Driving While Distracted

One of the big issues that often goes undiscussed with individuals with ADD is the role that their disorder plays in a very fundamental and basic activity, one that most of us take for granted: driving. Studies have revealed that individuals with ADD actually do have an increased risk for driving mishaps, including more motor vehicle citations and crashes.

While a majority of these studies are done on young adults, who are more accident-prone than older adults, certainly the distractibility, inattention, and impulsivity in any person with ADD could lead to problems with driving.

As we discussed earlier in this chapter, sleep derangement and excessive daytime sleepiness, which may be present in some individuals, may also play some role in the poor driving performance. Bad nutrition or lack of exercise could be additional factors.

In all fairness, other serious psychiatric problems were found in individuals with serious driving problems. In addition to their ADD, many experienced social disorders such as defiant or oppositional disorders and antisocial disorders. But even if your primary problem is ADD and you are essentially normal other than that, you can still have problems driving.

This does not mean that if you have ADD you need to take a mass transit or taxi and park your cars away indefinitely. But it does go to show that there is one more routine life activity that many individuals take for granted but which, unfortunately, people with ADD need to regard seriously as a daily challenge.

Certainly, most patients with ADD perform very well on the road, but, as one popular 1980s television show used to quote, "It's a jungle out there, be careful." This is no less true today.

9

Adaptive Devices for
Adults with ADD

In earlier chapters, we've discussed the use of medications, psychotherapy, and other methods and tools that people with attention deficit disorder can use to normalize their existence. In this chapter, we will consider various adaptive devices that can give the adult with attention deficit disorder an edge in their own unique Olympic games (challenging games of everyday life).

Although few of our readers have unlimited income—and we understand this—it's also true that there are a variety of tools that make good financial sense, and many are not expensive. The small investment made in many of these adaptive devices can go a long way in improving not only your business and social life, but your personal interactions as well.

There is a wide range of categories of products, and good particular products within these classes, and we could never hope to include everything available in today's crowded marketplace. We divide adaptive devices for ADDers into low-, medium-, and high-tech products, and discuss why such products can greatly benefit many people with ADD. (See appendix V for more information on the manufacturers of specific devices described here.)

Low-Tech Devices

Certainly, everyone has access to a pencil and paper. Often, if we just had pencil and paper at hand when we came up with a brilliant idea, we would be able to sustain that idea and act on it. What is even worse, patients with ADD will often jot things down and then forget to look at them, misplace the list, or think, "I'll get to it later." Despite these problems, we strongly recommend to our patients that they keep a $0.29 spiral-bound pocket notebook with a pencil available to them at all times. In this same category, we would include such items as Post-it notes, although we understand the difficulty in hanging onto these objects.

Another additional essential item under this category would include a small pocket calendar that can be used to jot down appointments, anniversaries, birthdays, etc. Keeping a pocket calendar on hand is often helpful, as our patients are less likely to be caught unaware of what event is occurring when.

> *Julie S., a forty-two-year-old mother of three, was diagnosed with ADD some time ago. Yet only over the last few years has she realized the value of maintaining a calendar. She stated repeatedly that she constantly missed not only her doctor appointments (we had noticed), but she would also miss appointments such as school meetings, parent-teacher meetings, and other social engagements.*
>
> *We suggested that she obtain a calendar, and she did pick one up and begin to use it. She then was able*

to plan her week in advance, knowing what time she could or couldn't make appointments, as well as what time she had to be somewhere. She was never again caught by surprise, finding out on Thursday afternoon at 3:00 that she had a parent-teacher meeting at 3:30. Julie would know in advance. Although this simple system was not foolproof, because occasionally she would forget to look at her calendar, she made much fewer embarrassing mistakes by using this simple adaptive device.

Dayplanner

To further elaborate on the concept of a calendar, some of our patients have found it helpful to carry a day/date planner, a booklet with many sections and also with many adaptive features in one. These usually include a day-at-a-glance, week-at-a-glance, and a monthly calendar, as well as pencil or pen and notepad. In most cases, they also include a small section for anniversaries, birthdays, and special occasions or meetings. In addition, they also have space to write activities to be performed, what most of us refer to as our "to do" list. These dayplanners can be very effective and can be obtained at a very inexpensive cost.

There are a number of rather pricey name brand dayplanners, but fortunately, generic day/date planners have come on the market and are readily available.

Use Your Checkbook

Many patients with ADD have one classic flaw—their disorder makes them ripe candidates and easy prey for each and every marketing ploy available. Our patients don't need a high-pressure sales pitch to convince them to buy. Just a gentle nudge and many times, the product is purchased.

One of the ways to inhibit this impulsive "buy now" tendency is to slow it down, and the use of the checkbook can help you with this. (Of course, you will need to record every check you write in the little check register provided by the bank. This is a must. In addition, you should balance your checkbook when you receive your monthly statement. If you can balance your checkbook on the day the statement arrives, you'll be less likely to forget.)

We strongly urge all of our patients to avoid the temptation to carry much cash. Instead, we insist they carry their checkbook at all times. Even a credit card makes it too easy to purchase items, many of which are unnecessary impulse purchases. Impulse buys have placed many of our patients in financial straits.

Maintaining a checkbook may be difficult at first, and certainly does require time. It also slows down the purchasing process. As one of our more affluent ADD patients pointed out, "I like to carry money. I don't want to wait in line. I don't want to have to wait even for the credit card to go through. Bing, bang, I want to be in, out, and I want to take whatever I purchase home." As you might guess, this patient has bought many products that he had absolutely no use for, and they usually end up unopened or unused, gathering dust on his shelf.

Using a checkbook also allows a patient with ADD to keep track of his finances, so that he can accurately make financial plans. We cannot stress this aspect too strongly, because having the funds to purchase other adaptive devices, organize your life, or buy a nice car or home, can make all the difference in the world to the personal and emotional well-being of a person with ADD.

Also, there is nothing that torments a relationship more than financial stresses, particularly unnecessary ones. Fights over money and extravagant expenses can end a marriage. This concept of financial responsibility can make a world of difference in the life of an individual with ADD.

Medium-Tech Adaptive Devices

Beepers

If you don't have a beeper, get one. One of the most common complaints of the family members of adults with ADD is their inability to find the person. ADDers do not only lose their own possessions, they can actually become lost themselves. This is why the wife of one of our adult ADD patients insisted her husband always carry a beeper. He had a tendency to get lost at shopping malls and could be counted upon to disappear for hours, even when running a simple errand. Actually, he never was truly lost, he simply got easily distracted by all of the "neat stuff" he saw in the various stores, and would end up wandering from store to store completely engrossed in various items.

Fortunately, his wife kept the credit cards, and he wasn't allowed to purchase items without her in attendance. He had done that previously and had ended up in trouble. Now, with the advent of various competing companies providing pagers, these items have become extremely inexpensive and have essentially solved this location problem.

The beeper also allows individuals to be reminded of appointments and other events they would normally forget. Beepers that convey text messages have become fairly commonplace, and this feature can be very valuable, particularly if the person with ADD is nowhere near a phone. Although a cellular phone is very helpful in this context, two-way beepers are now available, and we predict that very soon they will be considered commonplace.

Hand-Held Recorders

These devices are very similar to the notebook and pen, with the exception that they are usually small, pocket-size recorders, and are readily accessible. They can store information on tapes that can later be retrieved and rechecked. With rapid technology changes, these items have been reduced in price from anywhere in the range of $19.95 through $79.95. The only differences in the cost appear to be related to name brand as well as some technical features.

We find that most of our patients can do very nicely with just the basic model. Of course, there are some disadvantages; one must keep a tape in the recorder. You also need to make sure the recorder has batteries, and that you do not destroy the tape. Also, remembering to listen to the tape is a crucial aspect of retrieving messages and information that you want to act on later.

Voice Organizers

Take the concept of the hand-held recorder and press it forward one order of magnitude, and you have the *voice organizer.* One great feature of the voice organizer is that it specifically eliminates the tape, which often becomes lost, tangled up, or broken.

Voice organizers come in a variety of types, sizes, and price ranges. Keeping in line the concept of medium tech, there are standard voice organizers readily accessible through many catalogs, as well as one we have received with the trademark label "The Voice Organizer."

The Voice Organizer is very handy in that it not only allows you to record announcements, but it also displays dates and times that are important to you. In addition, it provides you with a simple way to create memos and reminders and access a phone directory. The Voice Organizer comes with a handy credit card-size guide to using the product. (Bulky, confusing manuals are especially hated by people with ADD, so you will find this guide easy to read.)

There are a few minor limitations with the Voice Organizer, such as the learning process during the initial training phase and getting the recorder to recognize your voice, as well as the moderately limited memory capacity. This device can store up to about ninety average-length messages lasting two to three seconds each. This limited capacity may pose a problem if you plan on using the device frequently with longer messages or over longer time frames. Nevertheless, another category of "mid tech," this seems to be a relatively simple and effective way of maintaining and preserving ideas that otherwise would have simply slipped by.

Voice Recorders Enter the Digital Age

We are very impressed with a voice recorder called *Flash-back,* developed by Norris Communications of Poway, California. The service and concept for this recorder is very congruent with the needs of most people with ADD. Although the Flashback was originally designed for business applications, we have found it to be particularly useful for our patients with ADD.

It uses digital technology, the sound quality is impeccable, and it is very easy to use. Flashback comes in a very well labeled box with easy-to-understand instructions, and is one of the few objects that we could actually work with "right out of the box."

We found that our patients with ADD can learn how to use this device in practically no time. It comes with a training tape and a very clear and concise instruction manual.

What sets Flashback apart from all other voice organizers, are the digital sound clips, using Flashback technology and allowing for storage of either 18 or 36 minutes on each clip. The difference between sound clips versus a regular audiotape is that sound clips are virtually indestructible and are impervious to light, noise, sound, and environmental exposure.

The luxury of recording memos, items, and thoughts for more than two to three seconds at a time can really pay off for the ADDer, particularly with business meetings and appointments. (We'll discuss this device further in our high-tech section of this chapter.)

Facsimile Machines

A home fax machine can make a dramatic improvement in an adult ADDer's life. Messages faxed to you from your office can be very helpful to serve as reminders for agendas, appointments, etc. The fax is also a very beneficial tool for "inspiration preservation."

Many of our ADD patients are capable of generating hundreds of flashes of brilliance in a single day, but unfortunately they usually remember none by the time they get home in the evening. Some of them have adopted the habit of sending themselves a fax as a reminder that will be awaiting them when they return home.

In addition, the fax can function as a checklist reminder; frequently the boss outlines tasks that need to be completed. The problem is that the person with ADD may recall these items for only a brief period of time. But with the fax, they can jot down a list, fax it on home, and have a permanent record readily available. That way, rather than just acting on the two to three items you actually recall, you can check with your fax machine and make sure you've followed all of the boss's instructions.

Another good feature is that many fax machines double as a photocopier. This can prove invaluable for making copies for friends and family of items and issues that need to be addressed.

Answering Machines

This kind of machine is an absolute must for every ADDer, in our opinion. First of all, it is an ideal way to keep track of your personal messages, as these answering machines can be used as memo reminders by simply holding the memo button on the answering machine. In addition, these devices are essential for maintaining a log or record of individuals that call, as well as maintaining those messages. As with fax machines, the ADDer can send home messages and reminders that won't be forgotten.

We often suggest to our ADD patients that they avoid answering the phone at all for certain intervals of time, especially if it's that time of day when they seem to be at their lowest ebb. For example, lunchtime and the time immediately following dinner seem to be sluggish periods for some of our ADDers, and we suggest they simply avoid answering the phone at this time. The answering machine can take the message and then, when they have regained their energy and stamina, they can move forward in an appropriate fashion and function at their highest level.

Answering machines also offer a bit of solitude and respite, allowing you to still have contact with the outside world while at the same time enabling you to be selective about who you choose to interact with. Consequently, it provides a measure of control which is sometimes easily and quickly lost for ADDers.

"Does Anybody Really Know What Time It Is?"

A song that was popular in the early 70s, by the pop group Chicago, asked a question that truly hits home. One of the simplest and most straightforward adaptive devices is the *wristwatch*. Yet it constantly amazes us that some people— with or without ADD—don't wear a watch.

We feel it is essential to know what time it is. If you know you have appointments, you can then be organized enough to realize how much time you have left to prepare for the appointment and to actually get there. But without a readily accessible wristwatch, you set yourself up for the classic syndrome of arriving "a day late and a dollar short."

But a regular wristwatch is inherently limited. While we feel the watch is an essential device, we also strongly recommend that you go one step further and enter the digital revolution.

This revolution has led to the development of enormous amounts of storage capability, even on a very small wrist-watch. As a result, appointments, phone numbers, birthdays, and so forth can be easily stored. Some watches, however, can be a little difficult to master. We find that although most adults with ADD are quite capable of learning how to set them up, many soon forget the proper use of these devices if they are not used on a very frequent basis.

Our very favorite of these devices is the *Datalink* by Timex. This enormously powerful device is so simple that it truly is difficult to forget its proper operation. It comes in a well-marked package with simple instructions. You actually can program the watch using your home computer by typing in phone numbers, appointments, and times for it to beep on your computer. The information is stored very easily from your computer keyboard onto the hard drive in a simple menu-drive manner. You then hold the watch in front of the screen and data is sent to your watch from the computer!

The Datalink watch does require a computer operating in Windows, but if you don't have Windows, this can be easily overcome. Most local libraries offer loan time on computers, and the Timex software disk can easily be used in this fashion. One caveat: the Datalink doesn't work with a laptop or notebook computer.

Datalink also has alarms that conveniently allow individuals to perform scheduled tasks such as taking medications, etc. One feature many ADDers appreciate is the hourly alarm that can serve as a temporal reality check and awaken the ADDer from even the most complex reveries.

We recommend this watch very strongly to anyone with access to a Windows-based computer. In fact, it's interesting for us to see this device being used so commonly now, particularly among many affluent executives. Although they can afford much more expensive watches, they prefer this "all in one" life organizer that they wear on their wrist that keeps track of virtually every aspect of their life activities, as well as providing a basic function in the form of telling time.

Cellular Phones

Now that cellular phone prices have plummeted, and there is only a nominal monthly service charge for using the phone, we are recommending cellular phones to people with ADD. The ability to stay in contact with their families has been a tough issue and the cell phone can help.

Although a beeper or pager can be effective, our ADD patients also need access to a phone or have access to respond to their pagers. Also, for busy executives, we find that once they do have an inspiration, if they have ready access to act upon this inspiration, often these projects will get done. Even if they preserve their inspiration through earlier mentioned adaptive devices, often times they still need that next communication link to move the project forward.

This could be a task as simple as making dinner reservations or as complex as closing that important business deal. Having the ability to "do it now" makes all the difference in the world to many of our patients. We make one cautious recommendation, however. If you use a cellular phone, make sure you always have two batteries, one that is constantly being charged while the other is in use.

Better Living Through Medication— But How to Remember Those Medications?

Our patients with ADD have told us repeatedly that if they could just remember to take their medications, then they would feel and act so much better. Yet remembering to take their medications is a constant struggle, particularly when you take short-acting medications, such as the central nervous system stimulants. These often must be taken three or four times per day or at specific times.

We've recently found *pill alarms,* which are basically pillboxes with a timer associated with them. They are set for each time during the 24-hour interval that a medication needs to be taken. If the pillbox section for that time frame is not opened when the alarm goes off, it cannot be removed later. This means that with this device, if you don't take your medication on time, you have to wait for the next "window" when you should take it. This also prevents people from taking too much medicine because they forgot whether they took their noontime pill. This unforgiving feature is very helpful for some of our patients and an annoyance or hindrance for others, yet it might work for you. While we try not to make our patients slaves to their medications and we try to allow them to have a relatively uninhibited lifestyle, sometimes medications need to be taken on a regimen and this is one mechanism that can be helpful.

For the most up-to-date device to help you make sure you've taken your medication (and taken it on time), the *Medi-Monitor I,* from Medication Management Technologies, Inc. in Rockville, Maryland, is a very exciting new product that includes many valuable features. This product, invented by neuropsychiatrist Dr. Bruce Kehr (who treats patients with ADD) and available in late 1996, tells you what medicine to take and when and also gives you a record of how well you're doing with compliance. You can download this record into your computer. Medi-Monitor I is especially good if you need to take more than one medication, whether it's for ADD, arthritis, or any other medical condition you may have.

High Technology: Entering the Twenty-first Century

In this section, we will discuss some of the more expensive adaptive devices. These may or may not apply to each individual reader, and you should review and look at these devices based on your particular needs, lifestyle, and personality. We are personally very interested in these types of adaptive devices, as we feel they can have a dramatic impact in our patients' lives.

Schedulers

Databank schedulers have been around for some time, but now quantum leaps have been made with regard to additional data storage, ease of use, and interactivity with other electronic devices.

We are very excited about one product, The *Aurora Electronic Voice Organizer VR-390*. This device has some voice organization and voice memory (a 90-second voice chip), and is also capable of storing thousands of directories and schedules. In addition, it has a calendar function, a timer function, and is able to store meetings, anniversaries, birthdays, phone numbers, and so forth. The VR-390 can function efficiently as a travel alarm clock too, and can be used by more than one person and with various voice mailboxes.

Probably most striking about this unit is its ability to interface by fax or modem with other devices. This means you can transmit information to others immediately. The device is relatively small, but still has an essentially full function keyboard, allowing full text messages to be entered with ease.

The design, layout, and utility of the Aurora VR-390 make it a simple device to use, once learned. We feel that this is a very important first step in a multisystem communication process, which often is also the most difficult step for our patients with ADD. Again, "inspiration preservation" plays an essential role and this is one very powerful device that can help in that role.

While there are other databank organizers and schedulers available on the market, we have not seen such a full function device with such clear organization as the Aurora VR-390.

Back to the Digital Revolution

We wanted to return to the *Flashback* by Norris and talk about one high-tech feature that really impressed us. This amazing device has the ability to incorporate your voice messages with a simple hookup. This means that with an adapter and a simple computer program, you can record your voice and transmit a voice file to your friend on the other side of the Earth.

We feel this is an amazing breakthrough in technology and is specifically amenable to those with ADD, many of whom are oriented more to listening than to seeing. For example, for many people with ADD, if they are told what to do orally, they can follow these instructions, while they may quickly become befuddled by printed handout instructions. As a result, we think that the Flashback is a device that was made for people with ADD.

The Personal Computer: An ADDer's Best Friend

For any person with ADD who can afford a computer, we suggest you get one at the very earliest opportunity. Just a little bit of computer literacy can have a very dramatic impact on the ADDer's life, and a computer is hard to lose, too. (You know who we're talking to!)

> *Felix S. was a salesman who was seen in our ADD center. He had only a very limited computer background. Since he could afford one, we recommended that he get a computer. Felix informed us after a few months of using this computer that the device had essentially changed his life.*
>
> *He told us that throughout his life he had the very annoying habit of losing documents, phone numbers, etc. After just a few months, Felix told us that his computer was his "information sanctuary" and that if he could just get his information on the computer he could always find the data again. He tried filing cabinets and other organizational techniques, but always ended up with "piles and piles of paper scattered all over the house" that was annoying not only to himself but also to his family.*

By having a source where all of his important information will ultimately reside, a "home" for his information, he was able to develop techniques that rapidly and fundamentally changed his organizational style. While he does not have the mounds of data in his head, he can retrieve them very rapidly.

Scanners

A scanner is a mechanical optical device that converts text or graphics into a computer-readable format. This means that what you scan will go into your hard drive or a disk on your computer.

The price of a good scanner has declined very dramatically in recent years. A scanner allows documents to be stored digitally on a hard drive and then placed in various types of filing programs or databases.

One of the programs with which we have had great success is *Recollect Gold* by MindWorks. This software package contains very powerful image and character recognition, allowing a very accurate storage of documents.

Once a document is scanned onto your computer's hard drive, it can be searched with this program by meaningful words. This program will scan your children's birth certificates, your fishing license, and essentially anything you can throw at it. A scanner and good program such as Recollect Gold can free you from the mounds of papers in which you seem to find everything *except* what you're looking for.

Modems

A modem is a device that links your computer to another computer via telephone line. This device can open up a world of endless information on virtually any subject. With a computer and a modem, it is possible to access the various online services, such as CompuServe and America Online.

By using these online services, you can access vast amounts of data from your computer terminal. It is possible to shop, make airline reservations, and do research on essentially any topic via your computer. Online services also have the various forms that allow users to exchange information on a variety of subjects, including attention deficit disorder. Information about other people's experience with medications, new research on ADD, and help manuals are easily available. If you have a question about some aspect of this condition, there is always someone online who will be willing to help you.

A modem will also enable you to access the Internet, something we regard as one of the major advances in human history. From your computer at home and at lightning speed, it is now possible to access computer databases and other types of information.

There are hundreds of sources of information on the Internet relevant to the ADDer. Many of these will be found on the World Wide Web. The Web is a global document retrieval system with text that is crosslinked to thousands of other documents that might actually be physically located thousands of miles away from the document actually being examined. Transferring from one document to the other is accomplished by the click of a mouse.

CH.A.D.D. and other ADD resources have web pages that provide information about physicians in your area, recent research, upcoming meetings, etc. Besides the World Wide Web, an important Internet resource is the UseNet Groups, which are essentially special interest groups on the Internet devoted to a various specific topics. Individuals interested in attention deficit disorder will post notes, which will be discussed or responded to by others who frequent this group. Information on medications, physicians, books, and so on will typically be posted on the service.

Even if you do not have a computer, these services will be available throughout the country with the help of a small converter box. The information will be transmitted via the telephone line or possibly by a cable service. You should also check your local library—some libraries are offering Internet access.

Electronic mail is also passed instantaneously over the Internet without the use of paper, complex addresses, and—the ultimate nightmare—postage stamps.

If Only I Had My Computer with Me . . .

As we mentioned, a personal computer can be a private sanctuary for information, as well as an access point for unlimited information regarding any specific subject that interests an individual. But home computers are exactly that—home computers. You can't carry them around with you.

However, in this age of miniaturization and microtechnology, we now have the subnotebook or the laptop computer. These are often extremely powerful computing devices, weighing no more than 4–6 pounds and can be carried in a routine attaché case. Indeed, we have set a number of our patients up with what we describe as a "portable office" with a subnotebook computer, a small cellular phone, and a small portable printer, all of which fit in a large briefcase and can be easily adapted to any travel style.

With this setup, particularly the interface of a modem and cellular phone and the laptop, our patients can access their home computer, get into their regular files, search through their home computer, and then download information into their laptop. This can then be printed out on their portable printer, or printed out on any routine printer device.

This two-way flow of information (obtaining information from a home computer base or transmitting information that is obtained in a business meeting to a home computer base) dramatically reduces the chances that information will be lost in transit and increases significantly the likelihood that information can be used to obtain a personal or business goal.

While there are a number of excellent portable computers on the market, we find some of the large name brand computers to be significantly overpriced for what they provide. Basically, our patients are purchasing a big name rather than a big function and more or better production.

Financial Software

While we already talked about a simple low-tech adaptive device—the checkbook—earlier in this chapter, certainly there are many high-tech devices in the way of computer financial software that make life very easy for our patients with ADD.

There are few things that a person with ADD hates more than income taxes and bill paying (not that people without ADD do like it). Getting your bills in order with the help of a computer is actually a very easy matter. Software programs such as *Quicken* can enable you to pay your bills quickly. Bills can even be paid on an electronic basis. Once the name of the payees have been entered, the amount of the check can merely be keyed and the check printed immediately. When April 15 rolls around, all of your income and expenses are very easily retrieved.

Personal Information Managers (PIMs)

There are a number of these personal information managers—software programs that record important personal information—which function as calendars, appointment organizers, contact managers, etc. The Aurora VR-390, discussed above, is one such example. Again, personal information managers simply absorb information input by an individual, and if it is stored appropriately and can be retrieved at will, they can increase productivity, reduce stress, and improve lifestyle in general for people with ADD.

There are also a number of software packages that allow individuals to organize their life through the use of increased computer organization with the information that is pre-sented. One such software package is *InfoSelect* by the Micro-Logic Corporation. This uses a series of topical display mechanisms and folders, is very simple, and allows quick and powerful searching of your data. It is extremely helpful in organizing ideas, E-mail, and essentially any type of informa-tion headache that you may have developed. Its simplicity and power puts it in a class of its own.

Personal Digital Assistants

Personal digital assistants are small devices that can be car-ried in a purse or small bag. They allow storage via the pen that comes with the device or by a small pen that converts your handwriting into recognized and storable information. Also, some of these have a detachable keyboard which can be used rather than a pen device, to enter information (New-ton, Zaurus, Pilot, etc.). Modems are available for most of these devices, allowing access to computers and online ser-vices through a phone line.

Wireless communication with some of these devices is available in many larger metropolitan areas. Information can be stored with regard to "to do" lists, birthdays and other anniversaries, as well as lecture notes and other items.

These devices are wonderful for "inspiration preserva-tion" and as reminding tools. The beauty of being able to send E-mail, faxes, and access online services from a small hand-held device can make this truly an empowering tool for you. We have tested the keyboard-driven devices such as the *Zaurus* by Sharpe and have found them to be somewhat clumsy, particularly with regard to data entry. Instead, we have found the *Apple MessagePad 120* to be easier and more convenient. Various peripherals will allow this device to send and receive faxes, receive wireless paging messages and allow access to online services in the Internet.

The *Pilot 5000* by Palm Computing is a relative newcomer in this arena. Not much larger than a traditional beeper, this very powerful device allows you to take notes, remember phone numbers, addresses, to-do lists, etc. When not in use it rests in a small cradle conveniently attached to the computer that permits data exchange between the two devices. This device will also learn to recognize your own handwriting fairly quickly. If it also functioned as a beeper (which it does not as of this writing), we would recognize this as a near-perfect ADD tool.

"Life Coaches": The Ultimate Adaptive Device

Did you ever stop to think of a *human being* as an adaptive device? Well, get ready for the latest craze in personal organization. "Life coaches" work in a variety of ways, based on which organization or agency you are affiliated with, how aggressively you want to utilize this service, and whether or not there is a positive response to this type of adaptive intervention.

Basically, for a fee, an individual (often a licensed psychologist or counseling technician) will contact you on a daily basis and, after an initial evaluation of anywhere from 10 to 90 minutes, will repeat contact with you on a daily or weekly basis. The life coach will outline areas in your life that you are working on, as well as areas in your professional life. Often, they will set up *manageable* to-do lists (not those monster lists that we all make and ultimately all fail at), and will check with you to see how you are coming along on your weekly list.

Coaches will also help organize a weekly, monthly, and yearly plan to help with meeting goals. While this is seen as frivolous and excessive for some, for others having a neutral individual interact in their life, even if it is for a moderate to expensive fee, can provide a great deal of reassurance and security.

We feel that, in addition to a formal paid assistant or coach, it is often reasonable to turn to other individuals to be used as "adaptive devices"; specifically, turning to a life partner or spouse and utilizing your spouse's strengths in organization, day planning, and inspiration preservation, may be helpful. Possibly most important is to find a friend with similar interests and someone who has technological ability, and simply "buy and do whatever they do." For example, if your friend who has some technology experience buys a Datalink watch, and figures it out, then you have an instant resource person to go to if you have trouble with organizing your Datalink. This applies as well to purchasing computers, VCRs, televisions, or any other complicated device.

If there is already someone you know, trust, and respect—someone willing to be the "guinea pig"—it is certainly reasonable for ADD patients to avoid "reinventing the wheel." This type of useless expense of energy leads to unnecessary frustration, financial stress, and, at times, failure.

This chapter has outlined a number of different adaptive devices, from those as simple as a notebook and pen, to as complex as a human being, and everything in between. While this certainly is not an exhaustive list of devices, these are many of the devices we have used with our patients, and they have had a great deal of success in maintaining ideas and preserving flashes of brilliance, and therefore our patients have been freed to act on their moments of brilliance, rather than agonize over their hours of frustration.

When it comes to the information superhighway, our patients have many ideas, and with the right tools are virtually limitless in their zeal to thrive in this brave new world.

PART

III

Other Issues

There are three important subjects that don't fall neatly into the categories of *identifying* attention deficit disorder or *resolving* it, so we've created a third section of "other issues." Many people with ADD have great difficulties in the work environment, so we're including an entire chapter devoted to coping in the workplace. In addition, relationships with family and "significant others" can become very strained when a person has ADD. We offer some helpful hints that we hope will help people with ADD both at work and at home.

We begin with a chapter on women and attention deficit disorder. Until very recently, women were essentially ignored when it came to ADD—a disorder long associated only with males. Only recently have the medical and psychological professions begun to recognize that women can and do have attention deficit disorder. We hope to contribute here to rectifying that oversight.

10

Women with ADD

We now believe that there are many women with attention deficit disorder (although it's very unclear *how* many), but it's been only in the past two to three years that researchers, physicians, and others have begun to recognize this truth. One of the reasons for this delayed recognition is that for many years it was presumed that girls rarely had ADD and, consequently, most research was based on males with ADD. Another reason is that many girls and women with ADD exhibit the *inattentive* form of ADD rather than the *hyperactivity* seen more frequently in male children.

ADD can have a very profound impact on women, perhaps even greater than its effect on men, because many times women are the caregivers to children and others. Despite our "liberated" culture today, in many instances the liberation is more like a hectic rat race, with women working 9 to 5, picking the kids up at the daycare center on the way home from work, rushing to fix dinner, helping with homework, and so on. All of these "must-dos," taken together, present a daunting series of tasks even for the average person. Add in the factor of ADD, and many women can definitely feel a "systems overload."

In addition, the expectations of others are very powerful. Why did Mom forget to help Karen with her spelling? Or forget to give her lunch money? Why did she lose that important paper for the class trip? Let alone the myriad of mistakes Mom can make at work.

Not a mother? Life's still tough. Let's take the unmarried woman, and let's say she earns a good salary, even has her own secretary to handle the daily details. She should be okay, right? Where this woman may fall down is in her personal relationships, finances, and the other areas where many people with ADD sometimes falter, slip, and fall.

Experts say that girls with ADD may have greater problems than boys do with low self-esteem and depression. It seems probable that we could generalize this finding to adult females with attention deficit disorder. In fact, in one study of girls with ADD, it was found that their relatives were at higher risk for ADD, depression, and anxiety than were the relatives of boys with ADD.

Other experts have speculated that girls with ADD who are diagnosed have a more extreme case of ADD than does the average boy. This may be because teachers and parents don't look for ADD in girls, assuming it appears primarily or solely in boys. As a result, only extremely hyperactive girls were seen as possibly having ADD.

Fortunately, physicians and mental health professionals today who acknowledge ADD do realize that the disorder can occur in females. In fact, it is probably more likely that an adult female who seeks help will get diagnosed than will a female child—basically because most parents are still not taking girls to be evaluated for ADD. This says little for our female children, but hopefully this problem will be resolved soon.

This chapter covers the primary *gender-specific* problem areas reported by women with ADD. As a result, problems common to both sexes, such as forgetting to take medications or hyperfocusing, are covered in other chapters.

Self-Quiz for Women Who May Have ADD

1. Do you lose things inside your purse—or your purse itself—more than once a week?
   ☐ Yes
   ☐ No

2. Do you need to return to your house or office more than twice a week because you forgot something?
   ☐ Yes
   ☐ No

3. Do you find yourself delaying projects until the last minute and then frantically trying to get them done?
   ☐ Yes
   ☐ No

4. Assume you are unmarried. You have a date with a special someone, but you can't decide what to wear. You change your clothes at least four times. You're late. Sound familiar?
   ☐ Yes
   ☐ No

5. Time to do the laundry. You wash and dry the clothes. And then leave them in the laundry basket (at least once a week).
   ☐ Yes
   ☐ No

6. If you have a child in school, you have trouble helping your child keep up with homework.
   ☐ Yes
   ☐ No

7. You want to go on a picnic. But on the way there, you see a sign for the art festival, so you tell your family that you will go there instead. At the art festival, you see a sign for a new restaurant opening. You cut short the art festival to go

to the restaurant. On the way to the restaurant, chances are good you'll be distracted by something else. Is this you?

☐ Yes

☐ No

8. When people praise you, you feel like an impostor. If they only knew how hard you had to work to just get by. Do these statements describe you?

☐ Yes

☐ No

9. When you were a child in school, other kids called you names like airhead, spacey, and so forth. You day-dreamed a lot. Was this you?

☐ Yes

☐ No

10. You find yourself blurting out things and wish you could censor your words better. Sometimes you hurt other people's feelings by what you say. Do these statements describe you?

☐ Yes

☐ No

If you have answered "yes" to more than five of these state-ments, you may have attention deficit disorder. Consider see-ing a physician who understands ADD for an evaluation.

Task-Oriented Problems

This section covers tasks that trouble many women with ADD, and the section that follows discusses emotional and relationship issues unique to females.

The House Is a Mess and You Are Guilty

Many women with ADD are clueless when it comes to house-keeping. Even a small one-bedroom apartment may seem as daunting as the Hearst Castle when it comes time to start scrubbing and cleaning. Why? One reason is they don't know where to start. Another reason is they forgot where the cleaning things are. A third reason is procrastination—not a reason we can necessarily attribute to ADD. (Who *likes* to clean?) Also, organization comes hard to most women with ADD, and cleaning the house is an organizational task. If you actually like cleaning your house, you probably don't have ADD.

Why is this a *woman* problem? Don't men have to clean too? Sure. They just don't feel guilty about it if they don't. One solution: do the best you can and just accept that as good enough. Are you June Cleaver from "Leave It to Beaver"? Is anyone? On the other hand, you don't want your house condemned by the Public Health Department. Find a happy medium.

Taking the Kids Everywhere, or Being on Time Yourself

Maybe you're not messy, but you're very distractible, moving from one task to another and having trouble finishing anything. Distractibility is a problem for men with ADD, but if you're an adult woman, you're expected to be on time—to the doctor, to work—everywhere. Certainly when you're taking your child to the pediatrician, you should be on time. (So you can sit there and wait, with everyone else.)

When you aren't on time, there are a lot of names that can be attributed to you, like "airhead," and so forth. If a man is late, that isn't good, but he may simply be "absent-minded," whereas late women are perceived as flaky.

And if you are late for—or, heavens!—don't even show up for some event at the local school, let's say a program your own child is in, well, there it is: you're a "bad mother." You're neglectful, deadbeat, negligent, you just don't care. Actually, you care a lot, but your ADD crowded out that information and it just didn't surface in time. Or at all.

One way to deal with the lateness problem is to write yourself little notes or to buy one of those watches that you can pre-program. (Timex makes one, called Datalink, described in chapter 9.) Some people leave Post-it notes all over the house. If it works for you, then fine. Use it.

Work Issues

We discuss work in chapter 12, but there are some work issues that are especially problematic for women (and they may cross over from task-oriented problems to relationship issues)—everything from not meeting deadlines to impulsively starting on a new and exciting way of achieving the mission. It may work and it may also aggravate everyone else who works on the job.

Sometimes work can be very stressful and a woman with ADD could blow up—or cry. One of our patients, Mary, had recently been promoted and now she supervised ten people. One day at a staff meeting, her staff began to argue about how to proceed with a problem. Mary hadn't slept much the previous night and she was also wondering if her new boyfriend was going to dump her because she'd forgotten to meet him for their date.

It all became too much for her, so she started crying, in front of everyone. They all looked discreetly away. Mary wondered if they were all heartless cold people, both males and females. Not really. Mary was the supervisor so she was in charge and her subordinates believed that to acknowledge Mary's emotional outburst would cause her to lose face. How could they take orders from someone who was acting like a baby? So they talked around her and ignored her.

There are a lot of advantages to being a supervisor when you have ADD, because you often have someone to make your appointments (and remind you of them) and keep track of your daily schedule. But the price is that you're expected to maintain an emotional equilibrium. This can be very tough for a woman, and especially for a woman with ADD.

Mary heard about ADD on a television program and made an appointment to see her neurologist. The doctor did diagnose Mary with ADD, as well as a low-grade case of depression. Today Mary takes Ritalin and Prozac and is far more even-tempered than she was in the past.

Women Are Supposed to Be Tactful and Kind

You probably really *are* a kind person—but we all have negative thoughts about others once in a while. The problem that the woman with ADD has is that she blurts these thoughts out. They may not even be that negative—they could be "left-handed compliments": "That dress doesn't make you look *that* fat." The self-censoring mechanism that people who don't have ADD use without thinking is absent in the woman with ADD.

Not that men with ADD can't blurt out remarks too. But men can often get away with insensitive remarks because they're, well, men. Women are supposed to be kind and compassionate and understanding—and keep their mouths shut. (On the other hand, you always know where you stand with a woman with ADD—she'll tell you!)

Sometimes medication can help you stop blurting out remarks, and sometimes it can at least blunt the tendency. But often women with ADD need to consciously work on thinking first, speaking second.

Relationship Issues

The key relationship issues for women with ADD appear to be problems with spouses or significant others, and with children. If your parents don't like the ADD, you can explain it to them, but there's not much else you can do. Same for your friends. Some people suggest making a joke of your chronic distractibility and impulsivity.

If you happen to live with a man and/or children with ADD themselves, your life is complicated many times over! But one thing is sure—life will rarely be boring at your house.

Dating Can Be a Challenge

Although men with ADD can have problems dating, women, again, are expected to be on time, composed, and so forth. If they're not, the man—especially a man who doesn't have ADD—not only thinks the woman doesn't care about him, but he may also think she's strange. The good news is that in most cases, the kind of man you want to date will be accepting of most of your foibles, particularly if you explain the ADD problem.

Sexuality can be another land mine for the woman with ADD, in part because of her impulsivity. Some women have been characterized as slutty or even nymphomaniacs because they choose to have sex with a man relatively quickly. Rarely is a man called a "Don Juan," despite how sexually active he may be.

Actually, in today's world, it really is a good idea for women (and men too!) to let sex wait until you feel you really know the person you're dating, and that you want to have a continuing relationship. (And of course it's always very important for the man to use a condom so you avoid HIV and other sexually transmitted diseases.)

Marriage Can Be Tough

Virtually every newlywed woman is sure that this man is the only one for her and their love will conquer any big or little problems they may have. One of those "little" problems may be that he is a neat freak and she has piles everywhere. Of course, all newlyweds go through an adjustment period where they learn to accommodate each other's daily habits. Or try to change them.

The thing is, she may not be able to get rid of her piles. And he may not be able to comprehend why not. Why doesn't she try harder? Why doesn't she have a neat room like his mom, also a neat freak, always had? (Maybe it's genetic is one answer.)

If *he* had piles everywhere, that might be annoying to the non-ADD wife, but men do stuff like that, don't they? Women are supposed to be neat, and if they aren't, well, maybe they're not so feminine after all. The stereotyping is endless.

Says Claudia P., "My spouse is an engineer and the exact opposite of me. This is not an easy relationship for either of us because he is neat, orderly, and on time for everything. I am always looking for stuff, always late, and disorganized. He finds me annoying and I confess I often feel the same about him and his anal-retentive lifestyle!"

What Claudia and her husband need to realize about each other is that his "anal-retentive lifestyle" is probably as much hardwired in his brain as is Claudia's ADD, thus they need to learn to be more accepting of each other.

An Established Marriage

Don't assume that just because you've been married ten or twenty or more years that your spouse will always understand and accept your ADD. Perhaps your spouse never knew anything about ADD until you were recently diagnosed. It's a good idea for the *physician* to explain to the spouse as well as to the ADDer what attention deficit really is and what symptoms in particular the patient has.

The doctor should also explain to the spouse what solutions can be tried, including medication, therapy, and various lifestyle changes, and also explain how the spouse might be able to assist. Of course if your spouse also has ADD, you already know that it's sometimes a very rocky ride through life! But hopefully one advantage to being married to an ADDer is that your spouse can understand and acknowledge the existence of attention deficit disorder.

The Kids Come!

In looking back, many couples say that before they had kids, life was fairly smooth, with a few wrinkles here and there. Afterwards, nothing is the same. Which is good and bad. Children need schedules, they need to be fed on a regular basis, and they need plenty of tender loving care.

Most ADDers don't have any trouble with the loving care part. But the regular schedules can be very difficult. Don't presume you have to be a perfect parent, but do understand that children don't thrive on chaos but rather on order. And trying to infuse order into your child's life may also help you to organize your own.

Said a mother with ADD, "I have two kids and when they both talk to me at the same time, I flip out. I can only attend to their needs one at a time, and it makes me feel like a failure as a mom. It's extremely hard to structure their lives, since my own is so unstructured."

So what to do? Experts recommend therapy as one help, and support groups can provide a morale booster as well as practical information. Don't forget to hire babysitters, too, so you can give yourself time off from the kids.

11

ADD and the Family

⟨decorative ornament⟩

*"No man is an island, entire of itself;
every man is a piece of the continent."*
—*John Donne,* Devotions *(1624)*

We've talked about many aspects of ADD so far, but now we'll take a more intimate look at the family role played by individuals with attention deficit disorder. By "family" we can include significant others, social situations, and relationships in general.

Our experience with patients and the responses we've received through questionnaires placed on the Internet and CompuServe have strongly indicated that family issues are very important to people with ADD. Perhaps the following comments hit a familiar chord. Have you ever said them?

1. I'm bored with my husband/wife/girlfriend/boyfriend.

2. They don't understand me.

3. They're always intruding at the wrong time.

4. They make me feel bad when I lose or misplace objects, although invariably I always find them.

5. I'm more comfortable doing things my way than other ways.

6. I don't know why I can't get credit for doing the things I do, rather than for not doing the things that need to get done.

7. I know I'll get to it, if I could just find the time.

8. It's not that I don't want to follow through on things. Rather, it seems like other issues always intrude and more important things come along.

9. It is frustrating when I make lists; I just lose the lists.

10. I'm not comfortable talking about sexual intimacy. I wish there was some way they could understand when I'm "in the mood" and when I'm not.

11. I've never asked him/her to clean up my mess; I like my mess.

12. I really don't try to make my life so hard, it just seems to always happen that way.

If any or all of these statement seem to fit, be reassured that you're not alone. These are common statements, and certainly ones we have heard repeatedly from sufferers with this disorder. We also hear from significant others, "Why can't he just straighten himself out?" or "She just doesn't try" or "He doesn't even make an effort."

As physicians treating this disorder, we realize that this all is not as simple as it may seem. As you are aware, ADD affects all aspects of your life, especially the interpersonal aspects, those affecting how you relate to a significant other, such as spouse, family, sibling, or coworker or even friend. In this chapter, we offer you some concrete, practical suggestions for dealing with others when you have ADD. And, later in the chapter, we also present suggestions for those significant others who are dealing with someone with ADD.

Suggestions for People with ADD

1. Communicate. This is essential. If you can explain this disorder, particularly to someone with whom you share a significant amount of time and emotional energy, help them understand that this is truly a disorder. This is *not an excuse*, but an explanation of your behavior, and a clear explanation will empower them to assist you in working with you to improve your relationship.

   As we have said before, it is best if a *physician* can explain the disorder to your spouse or significant other. A physician's analytical understanding, and more detached viewpoint, will help your partner understand the situation in more objective, clinical terms. This kind of presentation will help your partner see that ADD is not an excuse, but an authentic condition that requires treatment.

   In addition to explaining that this is part of your disorder, provide information to read, such as information from the CH.A.D.D. (Children and Adults with Attention Deficit Disorder) Newsletter. Let them read this book. Simply knowing that ADD is a medical disorder, not a "personality flaw," will help them understand that they need to work with you on this, particularly if they are invested in your life.

2. Take a neutral stance. What we mean by this is that this is not about judgment, or one person being right and the other wrong, or vice versa; rather, this is the way things are. Approaching the situation in a nonthreatening, nonhostile fashion, where one or the other individual is not becoming defensive, relates back to tip #1: communicate.

   Make sure that your friends and family understand that you are not angry with them, but may indeed at times be frustrated with their lack of understanding and patience with you. Help them see that with assistance you can change and modify your behavior.

3. The "Count to Ten" Rule. One of the hallmarks of ADD is impulsivity, reacting without predicting the consequences

of your actions. Instead, take a deep breath and count to ten. This can help to keep you from blurting out things you might regret. Whether it's your boss criticizing your work or your spouse complaining that she asked you nine times to take out the trash . . . count to ten, compose your thoughts, and *then* speak. (Or, if appropriate, hold your tongue.)

Incorporating this simple calming procedure into your life can mean a world of difference, not only in what comes out of you but in *the way* it comes out.

4. Organization is everything. We refer the reader back to chapter 9, on adaptive devices. The most important thing in having a successful relationship, whether it's play, work, social, or business, is to make sure that items that need to be done actually do get done. And also that the items with the highest priority get done first. Often with this disorder it is hard to prioritize, and follow-through is also a big problem.

By having your social calendar planned, with a day, week or month at a glance, having (and *using*) adaptive devices, and knowing where you're supposed to be, when you're supposed to be there, and *why* you're supposed to be there—can make all the difference in the world.

There are numerous ways to organize yourself, as outlined in chapter 9.

5. Figure out your role. In every relationship, there is some degree of give and take, and although ideally this should be an equal, 50-50 process, this rarely is the case. Communicate your wants, needs, wishes, and desires; let others know how you function best, and how you don't function well at all. For example, if you have a chronic problem with lateness, tell people so that they won't assume you just don't care if you're not on time.

Find out what you can and can't live with and make sure that this is plainly identified and known to your significant other. Don't set yourself up for failure by agreeing to live a role you can't perform; on the other hand, try to be considerate and compassionate when it comes to your spouse or significant other, or other individuals involved in the relationship. As we have said before, ADD is a designation of a disorder, not an *excuse* for inconsiderate behavior.

Do not place your significant other into the role of servant, dictator, or enabler. Yes, often the significant other will enable a patient with ADD to continue their inappropriate and ineffective lifestyles, rather than facing these issues and forming an appropriate way to deal with them. (For example, he or she might simply straighten up the room, finish the yard work, or complete the unfinished project just to get it out of the way.) However, someone who is truly helpful might point out ways to keep the room neat (closet organizers, hampers, shoe racks, etc.). A helpful person would also place limits on what he or she did for yard work (and maybe lay out the tools needed for the person with ADD) and also might provide an outline to assist with finishing an incomplete project.

One couple we know falls into the "Mrs. Doubtfire" type of scenario (referring to the popular movie starring Robin Williams). One individual with the ADD is constantly coming up with ideas, thoughts, or almost a flight of ideas at times; the creativity that comes forth from this individual is astounding. However, it is also exhausting.

Another important point which could be learned from the movie *Mrs. Doubtfire* is that it's not fair when one person does all the fun activities and the other person has to be the serious one. In this movie, Robin Williams's male character was someone with ADD and he was very creative, playful, and fun-loving. But at times, he was also very irresponsible, compelling his wife to be even more serious, more responsible, more hardworking, and more "Type A."

Indeed, the wife points out that she did not like the way she became in response to him, stating that she always felt like the policeman, the one saying no, the "bad guy." This is a classic example of how couples fall into destructive rather than constructive patterns. Proper communication will lead to identification of the problem and some behavior modification, through which the situation can be remedied. In the movie, the character with ADD learns how to use his creativity in a positive way, becoming not only a super nanny but also a more empathetic individual.

One of our patients was as energetic and active as the character played by Robin Williams in *Mrs. Doubtfire.* One morning, before 9 o'clock, he already had come up with twenty-seven new ideas and projects that he hoped to accomplish that day. Clearly, this was going to set him as well as the relationship up for failure. In addition, by constantly being put on the defensive, constantly having to say "No, we can't do that," his wife became the "responsible adult" in the relationship, never allowed to relax and be creative, never allowed to be fun-loving, spontaneous, or carefree.

6. Remain an individual, identify and preserve your free time. It is absolutely essential in any relationship to remain an individual and to maintain some independence. Our patients with ADD explain to us that they need quiet time, time alone to do their projects, even if they don't complete them. They need time to be on the computer, to do their creative writing, painting, etc.

One person we worked with liked to do gardening. Although the garden never grew anything, because it was never fully weeded, for this individual, gardening served as a combination of stress reducer, relaxation time, and quality private time. He was happy enough with the garden as it was, but unfortunately his girlfriend constantly asked, "Why can't you grow anything? Why doesn't our garden look nice?" and constantly interfered in his gardening time.

We finally had to point out that this criticism was inappropriate. Even if the garden grew nothing, it didn't matter, because the garden served as a form of therapy, solitude, and nurturing for the patient. After this was highlighted and identified, from that day on the garden was never any better, but it was no longer a source of stress and irritation in the relationship.

7. ADD is an explanation, not an excuse. We have explained repeatedly to all of our patients that it is inappropriate to use this disorder as an excuse. Just as a diabetic would never get away with saying, "I have diabetes, so I can't make my bed, can't clean my room, can't work on this project," no one should use ADD as a rationale for not getting the work done. Don't allow yourself to fall into the excuse trap. *Don't become a victim.*

8. Negotiate social situations. This may sound trivial, but social situations can have a significant impact on a relationship. One of our patients refuses to go out socially. "When I get in a group of people," he explains, "I'm distracted by everyone's conversation. I end up going home angry, moody, and frustrated, because I didn't really understand or follow any one conversation, and I feel as though I couldn't fit in." This has been a source of consternation among the patient and his spouse, as she likes to be socially outgoing, and enjoys this as part of not only her professional work, but also as part of her personal life.

   They've had many arguments about this problem, and it was only recently that they sat down and figured out why they did not go out socially together, and what they could do about it. They came up with a plan: if they entered a crowded room or a social gathering, they would step aside into a quiet part of the room. Or if they attended a dinner party, they would sit at only one end of the table, rather than in the middle.

This proactive involvement in "managing the environment" made a world of difference in their relationship. It allowed the man with ADD to concentrate on just one conversation at a time and gave his wife the social interaction she desired. It also ultimately led to their being invited out to many more social gatherings. In addition, the patient's mood at the end of these evenings was now much more upbeat, when in the past, as he said, he would often come home in a sour mood.

9. Be nice when you can. While this may sound simple to the point of being ridiculous, it's absolutely essential. Everyday life activities—including work, the stress of life's time commitments, as well as coworkers', employees', friends', and family's requests—can be quite draining. The last thing an individual with ADD needs is a relationship where he or she has to be "on guard" all the time.

Finding something nice in another individual in a relationship may only take seconds, but that positive reinforcement can last hours or even days. And, conversely, if an individual with ADD is in a down mood, learning how to express this to a significant other, rather than snapping at the person or closing off communication altogether, may make all the difference in saving versus destroying a relationship.

For example, pointing out, "I'm just out of it right now" is much more polite and effective than growling, "Just leave me alone," or, even worse, "I don't want to be around you." Positive responses can help solidify a relationship.

10. Relationship time management. Practice this daily. Pencil in time for your partner on the calendar or day planner. Whether it's a dinner, lunch, an early-morning or late-night scheduled sit-down and face-to-face time commitment, scheduling time together can go a long way in preventing problems from becoming insurmountable. After all, if a relationship is worth having, it's worth keeping.

What If You're a Parent with ADD?

It's hard enough to live with your own shortcomings, but having to carry them on to the next generation can be doubly hard. Assuming that your children do not have ADD, it's important that you allow your spouse to be actively involved in child rearing.

Your strength may be creativity, you may be the fun-and-games parent, whereas your spouse is the organizer and the time manager. This is fine, as long as you each have your roles identified. However, if these roles cause strife, it's important to go back and review the items listed above. Remember that your spouse doesn't want to always be the one to say "no" to your child and doesn't always want to be the "bad guy."

What if you have ADD and your child has ADD too? This is more difficult. Learning that there is a rationale and explanation for your behavior can certainly take some of the negative stigma away from your child. However, this is still not an effective cure for the child. It is important to review chapter 9 on adaptive devices, as well as our chapter on counseling, and behavior modification (chapter 7).

What If Your Spouse Has ADD?

You may have bought this book because you suspect that your spouse has all of the cardinal signs and symptoms of attention deficit disorder. What can you do to arrange it so that you are bringing each other closer together, rather than constantly fighting, pushing each other away, and having to make up for things you feel could have been avoided in the first place?

As you know from reading this book and from living with the person who you think has ADD, the impulsivity, lack of empathy, difficulty with long-term planning, and lack of comprehension of the consequences of actions are all hallmarks of this disorder. Therefore, even with perfect communication, there are still going to be times of strife, as there are with any relationships.

For example, possibly she told you at the very last minute that you have an important social engagement later that evening. Or perhaps she failed to inform you she would not be home for dinner, would be staying late at the office, or possibly would be going away for the weekend. Does this ever happen? Do you ever find out about things at the very last minute, feeling like you're always playing catch-up?

Here are some suggestions for intervention, to be *proactive* rather than reactive.

1. Work on modifying your partner's behavior. To do this, it is first important to identify the behaviors that are *problematic* in the relationship, as well as those behaviors that are *reinforcing* to the relationship. This takes a moderate amount of objectivity, because it is important to realize that there are two people involved in every relationship. Look at the way you respond to his or her behavior changes when he is in an "ADD funk" versus when the person is in a good mood.

   Once the behaviors are identified, it is extremely important to notice when he's behaving in some way you want to encourage. We call this "positive reinforcement," and it works on children and adults. For example, when he does a project and actually finishes it, praise him. Make sure that he knows how satisfied and pleased you are that he's completed a task, whether it's something small like doing the laundry or taking out the garbage, or a large task like completing the room addition. There is no task so trivial that it does not merit praise when he or she does a good job.

2. Set your partner up to succeed rather than fail. Don't plan ten activities in a day. Rather, plan two or three discrete activities or events for any given day, all of which can easily be accomplished in a timely fashion. If you have twelve to fifteen items on a to-do list, invariably none of them will

get done. If you limit this to two or three items that you truly want to get completed, this is "doable."

3. Limit social interaction and activity, and outside distractions in general. Clearly, like the example of the man who would not go out to dinner because it was too distracting, if you set up activities that involve many diversions, the chances of completion are slim. Rather, if you have a limited set of plans, there is a greater likelihood that the task or project will proceed.

4. Help your spouse with ADD. Form a broader base of support. While this may seem simple, ADD and its classic behaviors of inattention, impulsivity, distractibility, as well as secondary social problems and inhibitions, may make it hard to establish social relationships. You can help by explaining to friends and family the basic features of ADD. In addition, you can subtly signal to your partner when he or she's intruding or monopolizing conversations.

    You can also let them know in a nonjudgmental way when they discontinue activities before they are completed, including when they're involved with social activities (such as stopping a bridge game before it's over, becoming bored before the golf game is finished, etc.). You can help point out when he's drifted off, lost attention, and point out to others how they can help him stay on track.

5. Last, and possibly the most important thing, you must be not only a friend, companion, and helper to an individual with ADD, but in addition, you need to be your spouse's *advocate.* After all, no one cares more about your spouse than you do, or is better able to act on his behalf. You are not a parent, but an advocate, a friend. This is also a good way to remove yourself from the "bad cop" role you so dislike.

Some People Will Never Get It

It's important to point out that no matter how hard you try, there will be people in your social circle and perhaps in your own family who will not understand ADD, no matter how much you tell them or how many books you offer them. They may not believe that ADD is a real disorder, or they may not believe that you have it.

Your own parents may find it hard to accept, especially if they always thought you were lazy as a child and just weren't trying hard enough. To acknowledge now that you've had an authentic disorder all along would be to acknowledge that they made a mistake in blaming you, or that they didn't look closely enough. This is hard. Be sure to convey to your parents that *you do not blame them* because they didn't have the opportunity to learn about and understand ADD when you were a child. It is not their fault.

It is hard to accept that some people refuse to accept and acknowledge ADD as a valid diagnosis, just as it's hard to accept that you have this disorder. But the important thing is for you to understand ADD yourself, and for your spouse and immediate family members to work with you on this. If people outside your nuclear family can't or won't understand, then at least you will have tried.

Conclusion

The good news is that there are many ways a person with ADD can improve family relationships. We've discussed some of the key actions we recommend you take. You can learn other coping mechanisms by attending support group meetings for people with ADD, and even by joining online computer groups on America Online, CompuServe, or the Internet. By hearing how others cope with family problems similar to yours, you can learn and try new tactics for effective coping in your own situation.

12

Work and School and ADD

⟞⟨⟨⟨⟨ ♪ ⟩⟩⟩⟩⟝

The working world can seem like a psychological minefield for a person with attention deficit disorder. Even the most lenient employers generally expect you to be on time to work and to complete assigned tasks by some deadline. And even the most benevolent bosses will be annoyed if they see a pattern of lateness, unfinished work, and overall disorganization.

College is another environment that can be terrifying for the person with ADD. For the young adult living at home with parents, perhaps they've provided the structure and support you need to just manage. But away from home, living in a dormitory or apartment with others and with constant activities going on, the person with ADD often becomes overwhelmed. Researchers who evaluated students for ADD reported their findings in an article in the *Journal of College Health*. The authors wrote, "Some were experiencing severe academic problems for the first time and felt they were not capable of performing at a college level." The researchers found, however, that many of the students were coping, although they clearly needed extra help and support. Medication and therapy was instrumental in helping the students with ADD. Of course, older adults often return to college and can find the prospect of handling a full course load and a family at the age of thirty or forty can be very difficult for a person *without* ADD.

Fortunately, educational institutions are starting to realize that ADD is a real problem. It's also true that educational facilities are included under the nondiscrimination provisions of the Americans with Disabilities Act.

This chapter covers some of the major problems that adults with ADD have in the world of work and education, with an emphasis on the working world because for most of us, far more years of our lives will be dedicated to work.

On the Job

One of the most common problems of people with ADD is that they are in the wrong career field. If you are a person with ADD, it doesn't matter if your father and your father's father were accountants—you'll probably have a very difficult time coping with such detailed work. Some ADDers are adept at hyperfocusing, but not on the same tasks, day after day. Even if you are successful with your medication and find that many of your symptoms of inattention, distractibility, and others seem well under control, a heavy detail-oriented job is hellish for most people with ADD.

Does this mean you should throw away the ledgers and join the circus? This solution might work for some, but most of you will want a steady job that pays enough to support you and your family. What you need to consider are your own talents and interests, as does everyone else when thinking about a career change. You also need to carefully consider your biggest problem areas as well as your strengths. For example, if you're always late, then avoid jobs that highly value timeliness, such as anything requiring appointments. If you're a daydreamer, you'd better not take a job that requires precision, skill, *and* attention. Looking at your assets, are you highly creative? If you're skillful at drawing, you might become an artist, or if you're verbally adept, perhaps you'd be successful as a writer.

Whether you're thirty or fifty, it is possible (which is not to say it's easy) to change your career and segue into a successful new career and lifestyle. In the course of our research in surveying people online on CompuServe and the Internet, we found ADDers who are happy in jobs that allow for variations in their daily lives. One man was a freelance photographer, with constant changes of scenes and schedules. Another was a police officer, and still another a paramedic. A woman with ADD is a social worker, whose supervisor understands and accepts the disorder.

Although the sampling of about twenty-five respondents was not scientific, it did appear that there was a pattern that those who seemed happiest in their jobs had a chance to exercise their creativity and allowed for changes in their environments.

But maybe you feel you can't change jobs and you're locked into your present position, at least for the time being. There are ways to learn to adapt to the working world, even when it's a job that's not readily amenable or friendly to a person with ADD. In fact, the Americans with Disabilities Act (ADA) does require employers to provide for some accommodations. (See the section on the ADA later in this chapter.)

To Tell or Not to Tell Your Boss?

It can be very difficult to decide whether to let your supervisor know that you have attention deficit disorder, especially today when the media derides ADD as a made-up and overdiagnosed condition. That representation is not true, but many people don't realize the falsehood that's being perpetuated. As a result, you may be afraid to tell your boss, lest she believe that you are faking to get out of doing your work.

Some people really don't have a choice, because, for example, they may be subject to periodic drug checks, and a positive test for amphetamines would look very bad if the person had not previously told the supervisor of the medical condition and the legally prescribed use of medication.

Whether you're an attorney or a clerk, you may find it difficult to talk to your boss about ADD. One aspect might be that you want to be seen as competent and hard-working and not perceived as "handicapped." Yet, at the same time, if you want and need accommodations in the workplace, then you must tell your supervisor about the ADD. If you do notify the boss, then you are entitled to reasonable accommodations.

Work Relationships

In virtually any job, not only your supervisor but also your coworkers will depend on you to play whatever work role you're assigned. If you don't accomplish your work, they may feel (and possibly rightly so) that an extra burden is transferred to them. ADD is a valid problem, of course, but this fact alone does not mean that your coworkers will understand or accept it.

Moving from Job to Job

Some people with ADD have great difficulty holding down a job and will move from position to position. For some, the boss may have fired them but for many, they become bored with the job and just want to move on. Of course, this is problematic in any career because career progression requires the ability for the person to move upwards as he or she gains knowledge and skills. But if the person never remains on the job long enough to achieve that level, then they are inadvertently thwarting their own success.

With medication and with therapy, the ADDer who has a problem retaining a job can learn to develop the patience and stamina to at least give a job a reasonable chance before quitting.

Overworking

Experts say that some people with ADD will work too much because the world of work is the one place where he or she feels competent. At home or in other environments, the person may feel confused and inept at coping. The problem with living to work is that the person will miss out on important social relationships with family and friends, as well as depriving others of his or her company.

Your Work Environment

Although most of us can't design our workplaces to our own specifications, you should do your best to limit the distractions in your work area. Whenever possible, try for a small cubicle with spartan surroundings. Don't surround your work area with numerous photos, signs, and other paraphernalia. Keep it simple.

If you work for a large company that employs an *ergonomist* (a specialist in office layouts in relationship to what's most effective/productive for humans), then you may wish to ask the ergonomist if he or she has considered the impact of ADD and how best to accommodate this disability.

In most cases, if you need changes made to your office environment, supervisors will give you what you need unless it is very expensive or difficult to achieve. Some people bring in their own distraction-inhibitors. For example, one woman brought in a white-noise generator so she would be less disturbed by office banter and traffic in and out.

If you need an accommodation that seems reasonable to you but which your boss refuses to provide, you may wish to invoke the Americans with Disabilities Act.

The Americans with Disabilities Act

Passed in 1990, the *Americans with Disabilities Act* (ADA) was designed to protect disabled individuals from losing their jobs (or not getting hired in the first place) as a result of their disability. Employers are also supposed to make reasonable accommodations for disabled people. The ADA applies to all businesses that employ more than fifteen people. (The ADA also applies to educational facilities; for example, one woman with ADD told us that her professors allow her use earphones during tests so that outside distractions are screened out.)

What is a disability? As defined by the ADA, a disability is "a physical or mental impairment that substantially limits one or more of the major life activities." Attention deficit disorder can be considered a disability under the ADA, depending on the severity of the problem. *Note:* keep in mind that the therapist or physician who diagnosed you with ADD should have used the *DSM-IV* criteria.

One important point is that you must be able to perform the primary job functions, even with your disability. Nor is your boss required to remove all stressful conditions from the workplace; however, if accommodations can be accomplished, they should be done. One example is the case of *Kent v. Derwinski* in 1991. In this case, a person's developmental delays and emotional problems made it difficult for him to deal with people at work. The court ordered sensitivity training for employees and the supervisor was ordered to be careful and tactful in disciplining the disabled man.

Although most people with ADD are not retarded, many are very sensitive and some have such emotional illnesses as depression, bipolar disorder, and other co-morbid problems. As a result, the just-cited case is of potential interest to workers.

Another important point is that even if you are on medication which brings your symptoms under control, the condition may still be regarded as disabling. In fact, the medication's improving effects should not be considered, according to an article on the ADA in the spring 1995 issue of *Employee Relations Law Journal.*

A "reasonable accommodation" for a person with ADD might be to provide a white-noise generator to block out sound, or a regular list of duties. Your employer doesn't have to provide you a corner office with a view, but, within reason, should help you limit the distractions that are difficult for an ADDer to handle. (The court-ordered sensitivity training referred to earlier was considered an accommodation under the ADA.)

There is a broad array of accommodations that employers could make; for example, an accommodation could include changing your shift hours or providing written instructions rather than oral orders. Other reasonable accommodations could involve allowing the person with ADD to sit in the front at a meeting so distractions are minimized. Or allowing the employee to stand rather than requiring her to sit. You may work better with quiet, or you may work better with the radio on softly. If you do have your own office but there's no door, it might be a good idea to request a door, to block out distractions.

The catch to the ADA is that you have to tell your employer that you are disabled, particularly in the case of ADD when there are no obvious disabling conditions. If you don't tell your supervisor and then you are fired, you probably won't have any legal recourse. But if you have told the boss that you have ADD and then you are fired, after your requests for simple accommodations were denied, then you may have a valid complaint against the company. Keep in mind that you do not have to tell your supervisor *everything* about your illness, nor are you required to report on medications you take for ADD. Only aspects that could affect your work need to be reported.

Many employers have complained that the cost of job accommodations is too high. According to the March 4, 1996 issue of the *Wall Street Journal,* Sears, Roebuck & Co. has spent an average of $45 each to accommodate the job needs of 71 employees. This is dramatically lower than their estimated cost of $1,800 to $2,400 to fire an employee and hire a new person. (A Harris poll has indicated that the median cost of providing accommodations was $233 per disabled employee in 1995.)

ADA claims are common, and according to a January 1995 issue of *Business Insurance,* ADA claims represented about 20 percent of all claims received by the Equal Employment Opportunity Commission (EEOC) in 1994. The most common problems reported were back pain, neurological problems, and psychiatric or emotional problems.

Of course, this section is only a general overview, and cannot substitute for legal or governmental advice. For further information about the ADA, contact the Job Accommodation Network at 800-ADA-WORK, or the ADA Regional Disability and Technical Assistance Center at 800-949-4232.

Jane M. thinks that employers should take into account the strengths of the person with ADD as well as the weaknesses.

"We all have characteristics, preferences, and abilities. The person with ADD has some that may appear as limits or require things to be done differently. As long as that person is 'draining the swamp,' or doing what needs to be done, then be flexible. Provide deadlines and structure to make their life easier. Listen responsively. ADD can require that a person spend a lot of energy doing what is extremely difficult for them. If you can reduce the tasks that are difficult for them, their energy can be spent in getting real work done."

Going to College

If you are an adult attending college, you may also ask for accommodations for your ADD disability. Some accommodations recommended by Kathleen Nadeau in her book, *Survival Guide for College Students with ADD or LD* are:

- Arranging to take only one exam per day
- Arranging for exams with longer times
- Selecting classes with small groups (when you can) rather than those based in large lecture halls with hundreds of students

You should also contact the Office of Disabled Student Services at the college and learn what services they offer.

Other Government Programs

Some people with severe cases of ADD find it very difficult to obtain or to keep a job. Regardless of age, they may be eligible for benefits from the Social Security Administration. If the individual has worked in the past, he or she may be eligible for Social Security benefits and also for health insurance under Medicare.

If the person has not worked, he or she may be eligible for Supplemental Security Insurance (SSI) payments and for medical insurance under the Medicaid program. Keep in mind that there are income and resources limits for SSI—which means if you have an income and assets, they may make you ineligible for the program.

For further information, contact the Social Security Administration at 800-772-1213.

The person with ADD who has trouble holding a job may also be eligible for benefits under the vocational rehabilitation program within the state. Your local state social services office should be able to assist you in finding the nearest "voc rehab" office. You may also be able to locate them yourself by looking under the heading for state agencies. For example, if you live in Florida, look under "Florida" in the phone book and look under this listing for state organizations. Most telephone directories have "blue pages" listing local, state, and federal government agencies. Check your state listings.

Getting Educated

As previously mentioned, college, vocational school, or other training programs for adults can be very difficult for the person with ADD. One situation that can be a strain is test taking. In one case, a person with ADD sued (and won) the right to have extra time to take the Bar Examination to become an attorney. If you will need more time than you think will be allotted to take a test, you should inform the professor ahead of time. If the professor is unresponsive, escalate the problem to a higher level, for example, the dean's office.

The sight of students taking notes is a common one on college campuses, but some ADDers are very poor at note taking. If this is a problem for you, you may be able to borrow someone else's notes. Or, with the professor's permission, you may be able to tape the lecture and listen to it later on. In some cases, the professor will accommodate you with handouts, if you are most effective at learning visually, rather than aurally.

Because of the distractibility and inattentiveness features of ADD, it's a good idea for students with ADD to *get to class early* so they can sit in front, where it's hard to fidget without being noticed. Do *not* sit by the window or door, where every passing person will distract you.

The world of work as well as higher education can be difficult courses to navigate for the person with ADD. However, with good medical care, therapy, a plan, and a positive mental attitude, you can steer around many of the obstacles to your success.

Conclusion

A ttention deficit disorder is a real problem experienced by adults of all ages and is no longer considered just for children anymore. ADD can cause devastating difficulties in the life of people with ADD as well as in the lives of families, friends, and colleagues.

But with treatment and hard work, ADD is a disorder that *can* be successfully managed by many people. The first key is understanding that you have it and the second key is determining what to do about it. There are actions you can take to better organize yourself and there are tools you can use to help regain control over your life, including many practical tips and devices that we've discussed.

Don't give up! Knowledge is power and many achievements are within your grasp. Forget what has been said in the past about you being an underachiever or not trying hard enough or being "spacey." Now you know what the cause was and now you can begin to navigate towards where you truly want to be.

We hope that this book has empowered you to understand ADD and also to take the action needed to make you life more successful and rewarding.

Appendix I:
Frequently Asked
Questions on Adult ADD

QUESTION: My doctor has prescribed a drug for me that I think may be an amphetamine. We used to call amphetamines "speed" when I was growing up. I'm worried if I take this, I could become addicted. Should I be worried?

ANSWER: The drug that has been prescribed for you is probably Dexedrine, which is discussed in this book (see chapter 6, on medications). Dexedrine is a very effective medication for ADD and does belong to the amphetamine class. The duration of action is usually quite short, although the medication is also marketed in the form of Dexedrine spansules, which are longer-acting.

This medication is usually taken in the mornings. It may be supplemented with an afternoon dosage if necessary. The risk of addiction with medications of this type is grossly exaggerated. These medications are prescribed with medical supervision and typically withdrawn quite gradually if ineffective. As with any medication, the risks and benefits must be carefully weighed. If this medication helps you concentrate and function more effectively, the medication is likely worth the (potential) risk involved.

QUESTION: My doctor prescribed a very low dose of medicine for me. I know this because my friend says she takes five times the amount. Why is the doctor giving me such a low dose? I am very hyper, and know I am much worse than she is.

ANSWER: This is certainly an interesting question. As we have stated elsewhere in this book, it is often very therapeutic for individuals with any chronic medical problem to discuss their condition with others with similar problems. A patient with attention deficit disorder will have much in common with others suffering from this same chronic medical condition. However, many differences, or "variables," are likely to exist as well. One of these variables is response to medications.

Even persons with the same disorder may respond differently to different medications and to similar doses of the same medication. It is important to coordinate dosage changes, etc., with your physician.

QUESTION: The doctor first tried Ritalin on me, but it didn't really help me. Then he tried Dexedrine, and that didn't work either. Now he's trying Cylert. I feel like a laboratory rat. I am wondering if my doctor is competent to treat ADD.

ANSWER: It can certainly be frustrating to be in a position of having to try many different medications. However, the more different medications we have to try, the more likely that we'll ultimately succeed.

The principles guiding medication therapy are fairly simple. One starts a medication and increases it to the point at which there is drug toxicity or until a therapeutic effect is achieved. If at a maximal medical dose of the medication is ineffective, it is certainly reasonable to try yet another promising agent. The dosing of this medication will follow these same principles. The medications your doctor is trying are perfectly reasonable to us.

QUESTION: The doctor prescribed Dexedrine for my ADD. I think I remember that this drug can cause weight loss. Does this mean I can abandon my diet? If so, hooray!

ANSWER: It is true that Dexedrine can have an appetite inhibitory effect. But this actually can be a problem, especially in younger children and adolescents. We do not recommend that this medication be used for weight loss, nor do we recommend that a "diet" alone be the recommended therapy for weight loss. A successful weight reduction program will depend largely on frequent exercise and an intelligent dietary modification plan.

Ironically, controlling an individual's symptoms of ADD may be the best weight loss program of all, at least indirectly. As the patient gets his chaotic lifestyle under reasonable control, the weight loss will often occur on a "natural" basis.

QUESTION: I have a lot of trouble remembering to take my medicines and sometimes even forget *if* I took them. If I can't remember whether I took my medicine, should I just take it, possibly for a second time? I don't want to overdose myself, but I don't want to not have enough, either.

ANSWER: This question strikes to the heart of the doctor-patient relationship. It is absolutely essential that an individual with ADD develop a supportive and dependable relationship with the physician. Absolute clarity must reign with regard to instructions concerning the medications.

If there is a question regarding medications it should be possible for the patient to call the physician's office and get clarification with regard to the medications. As there are many different medications used in treating ADD, it is difficult to answer this question in a specific manner.

With regard to your memory, if you take your medication using any of the various "reminding" strategies outlined in this book, which can include pillboxes and alarms (which can even be in the form of a wristwatch), one of these tactics should work. This should not be an insurmountable problem. (See chapter 9, on adaptive devices.)

QUESTION: My friend did really poorly on a medicine the doctor just prescribed for me. I'm worried that I'll get the side effects she got. Should I be concerned?

ANSWER: It is important to remember that what works in one person may not automatically work in the next patient. Individuals respond quite differently to different medications, and the bases for these differences are, for the most part, unpredictable. For this reason it is imperative in dealing with ADD to keep trying.

Discuss your concerns with your physician and keep a list of things you need to discuss when you see them. In our experience it would be a very unusual occurrence indeed that your physician would not be willing to discuss medications at the time of the consultation.

QUESTION: My son has ADD, and the teacher accepts this. But when I told her that I have ADD, she just gave me one of those looks. Why is it easy to believe a kid can have ADD, but people think you're faking it if you're an adult with ADD?

ANSWER: There is a great resistance in society to accept ADD in adults, as it appears to many individuals as a legitimization of what society essentially regards as "bad manners." It is quite likely that this stigma will continue for some time to come, although we feel that as this condition is discussed in the press and other media, this bias will ultimately evaporate.

You should keep this bias in mind before speaking about your ADD or any other chronic medical problem. This is your affair and has very little to do with the teacher's ability to effectively instruct your child.

QUESTION: I know my husband has ADD; he has every symptom. But he refuses to talk to a doctor about this. What should I do?

ANSWER: This is not an uncommon problem. Forcing your husband to seek medical attention in various ways, i.e., by threats, pleading, ultimatums, etc., can lead to disastrous consequences and even failed marriages. Try to keep in mind that, in this context, time is truly on your side. As we mention above, we expect the stigma of ADD to diminish in the future, and exactly this stigma may be playing a role in your husband's resistance to seeking medical attention.

While you cannot prescribe medications for your husband, you might be able to help him deal with some of the problems he faces as a sufferer of this disorder. This should, of course, be done in a very subtle manner and should probably consist mostly of helping him remember things and organize his life. Keep in mind, however, that pushing too hard could have disastrous consequences.

QUESTION: I have three kids with ADD and my husband has it, too. I don't have ADD, but I am exhausted cleaning up, literally and figuratively, after them! What should I do?

ANSWER: We assume that you have seen that your children and husband have gotten medical attention. Involving the respective therapists in the project can be quite helpful. One of our patients who complained of similar problems developed a "domestic division of labor" program which she successfully implemented.

The individual tasks were announced clearly on an erasable board located in a prominent location in the home. After a duty is discharged, a check is placed in the appropriate box, and the results can be discussed on a periodic basis. Various types of rewards can be used effectively in this context, as well.

Keep in mind that you should not expect a revolution on the first day. People with ADD can learn and develop effective habits, they just need more help than others.

QUESTION: I am a woman, and I think I may have ADD. I asked my doctor, an internist, about this and she says that it's mostly boys and men who get ADD, so I should stop worrying. Is she right?

ANSWER: Women definitely can have ADD. The current concept of this disorder being uncommon in women is probably based on the somewhat different presentation of the symptoms in women as opposed to men. Women often escape diagnosis because they tend to have fewer of the most prominent "red flags," i.e., the symptoms of hyperactivity. You definitely may have ADD, and you deserve proper diagnosis and relevant treatment just as much as anyone else.

QUESTION: I am a woman with ADD and I am taking Ritalin spansules, which work well for me. But my husband and I want to try to have a baby soon. Should I wait until I get pregnant to stop, or should I stop now?

ANSWER: We recommend that medications in general be avoided during the first trimester. We would not recommend waiting until you actually find out that you are pregnant before stopping medication, as damage is often done very early in a pregnancy. This is a very important issue, and you should not hesitate to discuss this with your treating physician.

QUESTION: I don't like taking prescribed drugs. Are there any good natural remedies that I can take for my ADD?

ANSWER: In our practice, we encounter individuals who have an enormous, inexplicable phobia about taking traditional medications. While we are puzzled by this attitude, we try to accommodate our patients who demonstrate their wish to try "natural medications."

Prescription medications in this country are rigidly controlled from the early developmental and trial states through every step of the actual formulation of the drug. Your chances are good that you will get exactly what is advertised on the bottle. Of course, other chemicals are often present as bulking agents, etc. There are only rarely any problems associated with these.

Why chemicals in medications that are touted as "natural" are automatically thought to be safe is a very puzzling phenomenon. Many vitamins can have serious consequences. (For example, vitamin B_6 can cause a very painful condition called peripheral neuropathy if used improperly. Excessive amounts of vitamin A can cause serious health problems, even pseudotumor cerebri, i.e., a serious headache that can actually lead to blindness if used improperly.)

The antioxidant pycnogenol is often used by people who have ADD. Many patients feel that this has been very helpful with regard to controlling ADD symptoms. This is difficult to understand on a theoretical basis; however, the same can be said of many medications in common usage in traditional medical practice.

As you probably know, ADDers are very impulsive and susceptible to many "get-well-quick" schemes. We recommend caution with regard to trying these new agents and also the use of nonpharmacological forms of therapy as we have listed in chapter 7, including psychotherapy, cognitive therapy, and organizational strategies.

QUESTION: I see several different doctors, a general practitioner and a specialist. The specialist has diagnosed me with ADD and put me on Ritalin. But the general practitioner is very opposed to this treatment. I feel caught in the middle. Do I have to stop seeing one of these doctors?

ANSWER: It is hard enough having a health problem without having disagreement among your treating physicians. This is certainly a nightmarish situation. This is another instance where the patient really must be informed and accept responsibility for his or her own medical care. Obviously, getting yet a third opinion might be helpful in this context. However, keep in mind why the specialist was consulted in the first place, i.e., probably because he or she has greater knowledge about a specific area of medicine than the family practitioner.

We would recommend that you educate yourself about the disorder that has been diagnosed and examine your symptoms in light of your research. Keep in mind the primary objective in dealing with ADD: functioning more effectively. Even if you don't have ADD, many of these strategies will be helpful. While medications are not likely to be of any great benefit, we would recommend that you think more about results than labels.

QUESTION: Some people say that ADD is overly diagnosed. Is it possible for someone who does not have ADD to be diagnosed with ADD?

ANSWER: Attention deficit disorder is likely to be both the most overdiagnosed and underdiagnosed syndrome of this decade. It is difficult to say which of the two is worse for the individual. It is certainly possible for someone without ADD to be diagnosed as having the disorder.

You can safeguard yourself to some degree by being evaluated by individuals with experience and interest in this particular disorder. You should not accept the diagnosis or treatment recommendations from someone who does not have expertise in this area. This principle would apply also to receiving the diagnosis from individuals without these skills.

QUESTION: I have PMS. Do women with ADD have worse premenstrual syndromes than women without it?

ANSWER: Any time there is a hormonal change in the body, there can also be a chemical influence on the central nervous system, and menstruation causes hormonal changes. In the case of some women who suffer from PMS and ADD, it is true that there may be dramatic increases in the levels of distractibility and impulsivity, with the peak occurring at the onset of the menses.

In addition, we find that ADD can worsen for some women during pregnancy and sometimes they may be perceived by others as "spacy" or "out of it." This distractibility is due to the pregnancy and the hormones involved, and after the baby is delivered, within a few days the woman should return to her previous level of ADD.

QUESTION: After I found out I had ADD, I was at first relieved to be diagnosed. But then I felt really angry that I suffered so unnecessarily as a child. Does this mean I need to see a psychiatrist?

ANSWER: Your response of relief upon receiving the diagnosis is very common. Often this is an extremely therapeutic event and liberates the individual to make more reality-based decisions about the great issues facing any individual, i.e., parenting, education, profession, etc.

Anyone who receives the diagnosis of attention deficit disorder late in life will be able to report many episodes of humiliation and other forms of mistreatment that the individual has received as a child. The seventeenth-century Dutch philosopher Baruch Spinoza once said, "An intelligent man thinks of nothing less than death." While it is unfortunate that we will all die at some time, there is very little use in speculating about this. The same is true with the various injustices that one experiences as a child suffering from ADD; this happened, but it is in the past and one should move on. Settling old scores or even whining about them distracts from your main task at hand, i.e., catching up and leading a fulfilled life.

Appendix II: Common Problems Faced by People with ADD and Some Solutions

Problem	Solution
Forgets appointments	Appointment book Timex programmable watch
Forgets to pay bills	Hardware/software with reminders on bills
Piles of papers everywhere	Clear plastic folders Clipboards, paper holders
Loses things	Special place for keys, money, etc.
Difficulty starting projects	Set date on which project must start, a date very close to now
Difficulty sustaining attention on projects	Break project up into workable segments Use self-motivation—if I finish this, then I can go to the movies

Problem	Solution
Forgetting medications	Place them in work station Take at specific times, or tie to events (like meals) Timex "Datalink" watch Taking spansules
Low self-esteem	Therapy Support groups Note: increased competencies should enhance self-esteem
Depression	Antidepressants Therapy
Confusion about schedule	Hardware/software that reminds Dayplanners
General messiness	Therapy/"life coach" Maid Acceptance
Forgetting important things	Lists Personal digital assistants
Forgetting instructions	Keeping notepad

Appendix III:
Support Groups for
People with ADD

National Groups

Attention Deficit Information Network
(Chapters in Massachusetts, Ohio, New Hampshire,New Jersey, South Carolina, and West Virginia)
National Office:
475 Hillside Avenue
Needham, MA 92194
617-455-9895

Biofeedback Certification Institute of America
10200 W. 44th Avenue, Suite 304
Wheat Ridge, CO 80033
303-420-9202

Children and Adults with Attention Deficit Disorder (CH.A.D.D.)
499 NW 70th Ave., Suite 101
Plantation, FL 33317
305-587-3700

Future Health, Inc.
3171 Rail Avenue
Trevose, PA 19053
215-364-4445
fax: 215-336-4447
Internet: 74354, 654@Compuserve.com

The Kerner Clinic
155 Granada Street, Suite "O"
Camarillo, CA 93010
805-383-3141

Support Groups in the U.S., by State[1]

Alaska
Anchorage CH.A.D.D.
Tel.: 907-338-1491

Arizona
Adults Seeking Knowledge About ADD
(Self-Help group)
Tucson, AZ
520-749-5465
Internet: Ledingham@tikal.biosci.arizona OR
Ledingham@aol.com

Center for Attention Deficit and Learning Disorders
Sanford Silverman, Ph.D., Psychologist
7125 East Lincoln Dr., Ste. 214
Paradise Valley, AZ 85253
602-990-4474

---

1. Some groups do not wish an address to be published, and prefer that a telephone number only be provided.

Della Mays, Adult Coordinator
Tucson, AZ
602-887-0978

Families with Attention Deficit Disorder Support Group
Marcia T. Brehmer
1704 Palo Verde Dr.
Chino Valley, AZ 86323
520-636-5160

South Mountain CH.A.D.D.
Jeri Goldstein, M.C.R.N.
Support group
Phoenix, AZ
602-345-6622

California
Adult Attention Deficit Disorder Group
Melissa Thomasson, Ph.D.
Arcadia, CA
818-301-7977

Joan Andrews, L.E.P., M.F.C.C.
Psychologist, Support group (children, teens, adults)
Newport Beach, CA
714-476-0991

John Capel, Ph.D.
Sacramento, CA
916-488-5788

CH.A.D.D. of Alameda County
Kathy Schnepple
Support group
Hayward, CA
510-581-9941

Pat and Monte Churchill
Support group
Pacheco, CA
510-825-4938

David Hayes, Adult Coordinator
Tiburon, CA
415-435-0994

Kitty Petty
ADD/LD Institute
Mountain View, CA
415-969-7137

San Diego Support Group for Adults with Attention Deficit
Disorder
Support group
Amy Ellis
Roland Rotz, Ph.D.
Learning Development Services
619-276-6912

Milton Lucius, Ph.D.
El Dorado Hills, CA
916-933-5217

MATRIX
San Rafael, CA
415-499-3877

Karen Neale, M.A.
Los Gatos, CA
408-395-1348

Colorado

CH.A.D.D. of Colorado Springs (adults and children)
2712 Westwood Blvd.
Colorado Springs, CO 80918
719-528-1163

John Cizman
Support group, adults
3383 Madison Ave., Unit W327
Boulder, CO 80303
303-786-8112

Maxine Jarvi
Support group
2624 Blackstone Ct.
Fort Collins, CO 80525
970-223-1338

Don Lambert (adult support group)
8050 Niwot Rd., #55
Longmont, CO 80503
303-652-8087

Dennis Smith
Littleton, CO
303-790-2354

Harry Orr (adults support group)
6980 Pierce St.
Arvada, CO 80003
303-458-5675

Connecticut
Attention Deficit Disorder Institute
(Therapist)
131 King's Highway North
Westport, CT 06880
203-221-4710

Block & Stein/A.D.D. Associates of New England
P.O. Box 220
West Simsbury, CT 06092
860-651-1367

CH.A.D.D. of the Farmington Valley
Support group
860-651-3880

Liz Johnson, Co-coordinator
Moodus, CT
203-873-1733

Joel Shusman
Independence Unlimited
Counselor, Adults
2138 Silas Deane Hwy, Ste. 2
Rocky Hill, CT 06067
203-257-3221
fax 203-257-3329

Delaware
Lizbee Mahoney, Adult Coordinator
Support group
CH.A.D.D. of Brandywine Valley
Wilmington, DE
302-478-8202

Florida
William N. Penzer, Ph.D.
Attention Deficit Disorders (adults and children)
Psychologist
150 South University Dr., Ste. A
Plantation, FL 33324
954-475-1371

CH.A.D.D. ADDult Group
Support group
Orlando, FL
407-263-4222

CH.A.D.D. of Collier County #576
Support group
Shelley L. Bensield
941-263-6861
fax: 941-774-9371

CH.A.D.D. Hillsborough/Polk County Chapter
Support group (adults and children)
Tampa, FL
813-882-5310

CH.A.D.D. of South Broward/North Dade
Support group
Lora Mills
Cooper City, FL
954-680-0799

Georgia
L.D. Adults of Georgia
Helene Johnson
Marietta, GA
770-514-8088

Adult Attention Deficit Disorder Support Group
John Teach, Ph.D.
Decatur, GA
404-378-6643

Illinois
ADD-ONS, Ltd.
Mary Daum, President
Support group
Frankfort, IL
708-510-0501

Marv Meyers
Psychologist
Attention Deficit Disorder Center (adults and children)
64 Old Orchard Rd., Ste. 712
Skokie, IL 60077
847-677-8485

Bromenn Counseling Services
Psychologist (adults and children)
Ron Ropp, Rel.D.
702 North East St.
Bloomington, IL 61701
309-829-0751

Deborah Dornaus
Peoria Pastoral Counseling
Therapist (adults and children)
Peoria, IL
309-693-0038

Gary Hubbard, M.S., L.M.F.T.
Loves Park, IL
815-282-1800

Indiana
Abilities Unlimited
Support group
Bloomington, IN
812-332-1620

Support group (adults and children)
Ed Morris
853 Connor St.
Noblesville, IN 46060
317-773-9459

Don Walker, Adult Coordinator
Support group (Adults only)
335 Lucon Dr.
Iowa City, IA 52246
319-337-5201

Kansas
ADD/ADHD Education and Resource Association
(adults and children)
2110 West 75th St.
Prairie Village, KS 66208
913-362-6108

Adult ADD Clinic
Avner Stern, Psychologist
4601 W. 109th. St., Ste. 110
Overland Park, KS 66211
913-469-6510

Kentucky
ADHD Diagnostic & Treatment
Louisville, KY
502-637-3022

Lee Epstein
Attention Deficit Disorder (adults and children)
Psychologist
3333 Bardstown Rd.
Louisville, KY 40218
502-459-7433

Nancy Blakley, Adult Coordinator
Support group
Lexington, KY
606-273-6772

Louisiana
River Parish CH.A.D.D.
Support group
Wanda Bardwell-Seiffert
Kenner, LA
504-467-4983

Maine
The ADD Adult Support Group
Lindy Botton, Larry Gilbert
Freeport, ME
207-865-3925

Maryland
Montgomery County CH.A.D.D.
Support group
Gaithersburg, MD
301-869-3628

Massachusetts
Linda Greenwood
Plymouth, MA
508-747-2179

Linda Rose
Therapist
P.O. Box 3472
Peabody, MA 01961

North Shore Adults and Children with ADD
Support group
Lynn, MA
617-599-6818

Lori Ray, Adult Coordinator
Greenfield, MA
413-773-5545

Michigan
David Maiseloff, Executive Director
ADHD Institute of Michigan
(children, adolescents, adults)
30161 Southfield Rd., Ste. 201
Southfield, MI 48076
810-540-9233

Adult ADD Support Group
Jennifer Bramer, Therapist
P.O. Box 40010
Lansing, MI 48901-7210
517-483-1184
517-669-9740

ADDult Information Exchange Network
Jim Reisinger
Dexter, MI
313-426-1659

Eastepointe ADHD Support Group
Detroit, MI
810-447-2845

Minnesota
Adult ADD Support Group
William Ronane, LICSW and John Matula
12450 Wayzata, Ste. 223
Minneapolis, MN 55426
612-933-3460
612-920-5535

Missouri
Attention Deficit Disorder Association of Missouri
Barb Rosenfeld, Adult Coordinator
St. Louis, MO
314-963-4655

Montana
ADHD Clinic of Montana
(Physician)
Great Falls, MT
406-453-6325

CH.A.D.D. of the Flathead Valley
Support group
Kalispell, MT
406-756-6159

New Hampshire
Adult ADD Support group
Sarah Brophy, Ph.D.
Concord, NH
603-224-4153

White Mountain AD-IN (adults)
Joanne Duncan, Coordinator
North Conway, NH
603-356-2714
603-356-2863

New Jersey
Adult ADD
Robert LoPresti, Ph.D.
Red Bank, NJ
908-842-4553

New Mexico
Robert L. Gurnee, Manager, ADD Child and Family Center
Attention Deficit Disorder Clinic
Psychologist
Albuquerque, NM
505-243-9600

New York
Attention Deficit Disorder Center
William Oldfield, Psychologist
Buffalo, NY
716-838-2811

CH.A.D.D. of Mohawk Valley
Janice Hall
Support group
Utica, NY
315-724-4233

CH.A.D.D. of Westchester County
Support group
Brewster, NY
914-278-3020

Greater Rochester Attention Deficit Disorder Association
(GRADDA)
Support group
Rochester, NY
716-251-2322

Susan G. Salit, M.S.W. Adult Coordinator
Scarsdale, NY
914-472-2935

Charlotte Tomaino, Ph.D.
White Plains, NY
914-949-4055

Ohio
A.S.K. About ADD
Support group
Bettylou Huber
Spring Valley, OH
513-862-4573

Attention Deficit Disorder
Support group
P.O. Box 198065
Cincinatti, OH 44512
513-241-4089

Oregon
ADDVENTURES Support Group
Portland, OR
503-452-5666

Pennsylvania
The Hahnemann Hospital Adult ADD Support Group
Susan Sussman, M.Ed.
Lafayette Hill, PA
610-825-8572

Dr. Tim Murphy & Associates (adults and children)
Psychologist
607 Washington St., Ste 403
Pittsburgh, PA 15228
412-531-4566

Southwest Pennsylvania CH.A.D.D. Network
Adult ADD Support Group
Dormont, PA
412-531-4554

Rhode Island
Rhode Island ADDult Support Group
(Age 18 and over)
Austin Donnelly, Director
260 Algonquin Dr.
Warwick, RI 02888
401-463-8778

South Carolina
Adult ADD Support Group
Ron A. Ralph
c/o Mental Health Association in Mid-Carolina
Columbia, SC
803-733-5425

Tennessee
ADD's Up (adults and children)
Support group
P.O. Box 120173
Nashville, TN 37212
615-292-5947

Texas
Central Houson Chapter for ADD/ADHD Adults
Chris Kipple
Support group
Houston, TX
713-521-2420

Dallas Chapter for ADD/ADHD Adults
Support group
Melissa Petty
12345 Jones Rd., Ste. 287
Dallas, TX 77077
214-455-3720

North Houston Chapter for ADD/ADHD Adults
Support group
Karen Kasper
713-353-3898

West Houston Chapter for ADD/ADHD Adults
Support group
Katrina Ricketts
713-870-0191

Utah
L.D.A. of Utah
Support group
Joyce Otterstrom
Salt Lake City, UT
801-355-2881

Virginia
Arlington/Alexandria CH.A.D.D. (children, adults)
Potomac of Virginia
5315 N. 16th Rd.
Arlington, VA 22205
703-536-6846

CH.A.D.D. of Central Virginia
Support group
Richmond, VA
804-254-0124

Northern Virginia Adult ADD Support Group
Susan Biggs, Ed.D.
Merrifield, VA
703-641-5451

Tidewater CH.A.D.D.
Support group
Princess Anne, VA
804-430-3673

Washington
Adult ADD Association
Support group
Lisa Poast
1225 East Sunset Dr.
Bellingham, WA 98226
360-647-6681

Attention Deficit Disorder Clinic
Olympia, WA
360-754-4801

Ron Jones
Attention Deficit Disorder Clinic
Olympia, WA
206-754-4801

Kathy Van Dyke
Kennewick, WA
509-734-9645

Wisconsin
ADHD Clinic (children and adults)
Debbie Fueger, Manager
Psychologist: Dr. Keith Bauer
10625 West N. Ave., Ste. 200
Milwaukee, WI 53226
414-774-9677

Adult ADHD Support Group
ADHD Women's Support Group
Paul Rembas
Waukesha, WI
414-542-6694

Robert Fuller, Facilitator
P.O. Box 8
Cedarburg, WI 53012
414-377-6900

Robert Lintereur, Facilitator
507-A Lake Bluff Rd.
Theinsville, WI 53092
414-242-5387

Online Organizations

America Online
CompuServe

Internet Groups

Children and Adults with Attention Deficit Disorder
(CH.A.D.D.)
http://www.chadd.org
Usenet group: alt.support.attn-deficit

Other usenet groups on the Internet that discuss ADD:
alt. support. depress
alt.psychology.pers
soc.support.depress
Also, look for Sudderth and Kandel's World Wide Web
sites: migraines.com and neurologist.com

Appendix IV:
ADD Checklist of Adult Symptoms*

—◁⫘〰⫘▷—

Do you have any of the following problems? Answer Yes or No to these questions, to help you in screening whether or not you may have ADD. (A professional evaluation is important.)

	Yes	No
1. Difficulty fulfilling work demands		
2. Difficulty working independently		
3. Has experienced frequent job changes		
4. Poor work record		
5. Difficulty organizing work-related tasks		
6. Difficulty organizing household-related tasks		
7. Low self-esteem		
8. Frequently shifts from one task to another before completion		

* This checklist is reproduced with the permission of its creator, Loren L. Hoffman, Ph.D., Neuropsychological Associates, Inc., Naples, Florida.

	Yes	No

9. Difficulty performing tasks alone

10. Engages in physically daring activities (skydiving, others)

11. Often impatient

12. Difficulty maintaining friendships

13. Difficulty delaying gratification

14. Difficulty sustaining attention

15. Impulsively acting without thinking

16. Overactive (hyperactive)

17. Unaware of future consequences of present actions

18. Attended college

19. Graduated from college

20. Difficulty with memory or learning

21. Frequent use of alcohol, marijuana, or cocaine

22. Trouble with law

23. History of frequent traffic violations (more than once a year)

24. History of frequent motor vehicle accidents (more than once a year)

25. History of depression

26. History of anxiety

27. Family history of ADD or ADD symptoms

28. Has a child diagnosed with ADD

29. Frequently confuses directions or gets lost on trips

30. Difficulty in school as a child and teenager

If you've answered Yes to eight or more of these questions, then you may have ADD and should see a qualified physician.

Appendix V:
Adaptive Devices

**Aurora Voice Organizer
  VR-390**
Aurora Corporation of America
3500 Challenger Street
Torrance, CA 90503
310-793-5650

Flashback
Norris Communications
12725 Stowe Drive
Poway, CA 92064
619-679-1504

InfoSelect
Micro Logic Corp.
P.O. Box 70
Hackensack, NJ 07602
800-342-5930 ext. 112

Medi-Monitor 1
Medication Management
  Technologies, Inc.
5920 Hubbard Drive
Rockville, MD 20852
301-984-1566

Pilot 1000
U.S. Robotics Palm Computing Division
4410 El Camino Real, Suite 180
Los Altos, CA 94022
800-881-7256

Quicken
Intuit
P.O. Box 3014
Menlo Park, CA 94026
415-322-0573

Recollect Gold Software
MindWorks Corporation
349 Cobalt Way
Sunnyvale, CA 94086
408-730-2100

Timex Datalink
Timex
P.O. Box 310
Middlebury, CT 06762-0310
203-573-5000

Sharp Zaurus
Sharp Electronics Corporation
Sharp Plaza
Mahwha, NJ 07430
800-BE-SHARP

Voice Organizer
Voice Powered Technology
15260 Ventura Boulevard,
   Suite 2200
Sherman Oaks, CA 91403
800-255-2310

Bibliography

Abikoff, H. "Cognitive Training in ADHD Children: Less to it than Meets the Eye," *Journal of Learning Disabilities,* v. 24, pp. 205–209.

Adamec, Christine. *How to Live with a Mentally Ill Person: A Handbook of Day-to-Day Strategies.* (New York: Wiley, 1996.)

Adler, Leonard A., et al. "Open Label Trial of Venlafaxine in Adults with Attention Deficit Disorder," *Psychopharmacology Bulletin,* v. 31, n. 4., 1995, pp. 785–788.

Alberts-Corush, Jody, Firestone, Philip, and Goodman, John T. "Attention and Impulsivity Characteristics of the Biological and Adoptive Parents of Hyperactive and Normal Control Children," *American Journal of Orthopsychiatry,* July 1986, v. 56, n. 3, pp. 413–423.

Arnold, L. E. "Nontraditional Psychosocial Treatments for Children and Adolescents: Critique and Proposed Screening Principles," *Journal of Abnormal Child Psychology,* Feb. 1995, v. 23, n. 1, p. 125 (16).

Baren, Martin. "What ADD Is—and Isn't," *Patient Care,* Dec. 15, 1995, v. 29, n. 20, p. 56 (14).

Barkley, R. A., et al. "Driving Related Risks and Outcomes of Attention Deficit Hyperactivity Disorder in Adolescents and Young Adults: A 3–5 Year Follow-Up Survey," *Pediatrics,* Aug. 1993, v. 92, n. 2, p. 212 (6).

Barkley, Russell A. *Taking Charge of ADHD: The Complete Authoritative Guide for Parents.* (New York: Guilford, 1995.)

Barry, C. A., et al. "Girls with Attention Deficit Disorder: A Silent Minority?: A Report on Behavioral and Cognitive Characteristics," *Pediatrics,* Nov. 1985, v. 76, n. 5, p. 801 (9).

Baskys, A. and Remington, G., eds. *Brain Mechanisms and Psychotropic Drugs.* (Boca Raton, Fla.: CRC Press, 1996.)

Bawden, Julie. "Diagnosis and Treatment," *Los Angeles Times,* Aug. 9, 1995.

Bellak, Leopold, et al. "Attention Deficit Hyperactivity Disorder in Adults," *Clinical Therapeutics,* v. 14, n. 2, 1992, pp. 138–146.

Bender, K.J. "ADHD Treatment Mainstays Extend from Childhood to Adulthood." "ADHD Special Challenges with Adolescents and Young Adults." Symposium material presented at the 8th Annual U.S. Psychiatric and Mental Health Congress, New York, Nov. 1995.

Benjamin, Jonathan, et al. "Population and Familial Association Between the D4 Dopamine Receptor Gene and Measures of Novelty Seeking," *Nature Genetics,* v. 12, Jan. 1996, p. 81–84.

Bennett, Robert. "Pharmaceutical Care of Patients with Diabetes," *Chain Drug Review,* Aug. 28, 1995, v. 17, n. 16, PRX 33 (6).

Biederman, J., et al. "Co-Morbidity of Attention Deficit Hyperactivity Disorder with Conduct, Depressive, Anxiety and other Disorders," *American Journal of Psychiatry,* v. 148, n. 5, May 1991, pp. 564–576.

Biederman, J., et al. "Familial Association Between Attention Deficit Disorder and Anxiety Disorders," *American Journal of Psychiatry,* 1991, v. 148, pp. 251–256.

Biederman, J., et al. "No Confirmation of Geschwind's Hypothesis of Associations Between Reading Disability, Immune Disorders and Motor Preference in ADHD," *Journal of Abnormal Child Psychology,* Oct. 1995, v. 23, n. 4, pp. 545–552.

Blum, Kenneth, et al. "Reward Defiency Syndrome," *American Scientist,* March-April 1996, v.84, p. 132–136.

Biederman, J., et al. "Patterns of Psychiatric Co-Morbidity, Cognition and Psychosocial Functioning in Adults with Attention Deficit Hyperactivity Disorder," *American Journal of Psychiatry,* v. 150, 1993, pp. 1792–1798.

Biederman, J., et al. "Psychoactive Substance Use Disorders in Adults with Attention Deficit Hyperactivity Disorder: Effects of ADHD and Psychiatric Co-Morbidity," *American Journal of Psychiatry,* Nov. 1995, v. 152, n. 11, pp. 1652–1658.

Bond, E. T., et al. "Postencephalitic Behavior Disorders: A Ten Year Review of the Franklin School," American Psychiatric Association 91st Annual Meeting, May 13–17, 1935, Washington, D.C.

Bond, Earl D., and Smith, Lauren H. "Post Encephalitic Behavior Disorders," *The American Journal of Psychiatry,* 1935, v. 92, p. 17.

Bordwin, Milton. "ADA: The Americans With and Without Disabilities Act," *Management Review,* May 1995, v.84, n.5, p.53(4).

Brown, Thomas E. "Attention Deficit Disorders Without Hyperactivity," *Chadder,* Spring/Summer, 1993, pp. 8–10.

The Brown University Child and Adolescent Behavior Letter, "Childhood ADHD Can Be Retrospectively Diagnosed in Adults," v.9, n.11, Nov. 1993, pp. 1–2.

The Brown University Child and Adolescent Behavior Letter, "Thyroid Deficiency Linked to Hyperactivity Disorder," May 1993, v. 9, n. 5, p. 5.

The Brown University Child and Adolescent Behavior Letter, "Urinary Catecholamines in ADHD with Anxiety," Aug. 1995, v.11, n.8, p. 6.

Brucker-Davis, F., et al. "Genetic and Clinical Features of 42 Kindreds with Resistance to Thyroid Hormone." The National Institutes of Health Perspective Study. *Annals of Internal Medicine,* Oct. 15, 1995, v. 123, n. 8, pp. 572–83.

Bussing, Regina, et al. "Relationship Between Behavioral Problems and Unintentional Injuries in U.S. Children: Findings of the 1988 National Health Interview Survey," *Archives of Pediatrics and Adolescent Medicine,* Jan. 1996, v. 150, n.1, p. 50 (7).

CH.A.D.D. "Americans with Disabilities Act and Its Impact for People with ADD," *Challenge,* Winter 1995.

CH.A.D.D. "Controversial Treatments for Children with ADD." *CHADD Facts #6,* 1993.

CH.A.D.D. "Parenting a Child with Attention Deficit Disorder." *CH.A.D.D. Facts #2,* 1993.

Chisholm, Patricia. "The ADD Dilemma: Is Ritalin the Best Way to Treat Attention Deficit Disorder?" *McLeans,* March 11, 1996, v. 109, n. 11, p. 42 (3).

Ciaranello, D. "Attention Deficit Hyperactivity Disorder and Resistance of Thyroid Hormone—A New Idea," *New England Journal of Medicine,* April 8, 1993, v. 328, n. 14, p. 1038 (2).

CKG. "SPECT Imaging Abnormalities in Attention Deficit Hyperactivity Disorder," *Clinical Nuclear Medicine,* v. 20, n. 1,1995, pp. 55–60.

Cocores, James A., et al. "Brief Communication: Cocaine Abuse, Attention Deficit Disorder, and Bipolar Disorder," *The Journal of Nervous and Mental Disease,* v. 175, 1987, pp. 431–432.

Cook, Edwin H., et al. "Association of Attention Deficit Disorder and the Dopamine Transporter Gene," *American Journal of Human Genetics,* v. 56, 1995, pp. 993–998.

Cramond, Bonnie. "Attention Deficit Hyperactivity Disorder and Creativity—What is the Connection?," *The Journal of Creative Behavior,* v. 28, n. 3, 3rd quarter, 1994.

Daly, J. M., Fritsch, S. L. "Case Study: Residual Attention Deficit Disorder Associated with Failure to Thrive in a Two-Month-Old Infant," *Journal of American Academy of Child and Adolescence,* 1995; v. 34, n. 1, pp. 55–57.

Denckla, M. B. "The Child with Developmental Disabilities Grown-Up: Adult Residual of Childhood Disorders," *Neurologic Clinics,* v. 11, n. 1, Feb. 1993, pp. 105–125.

Denckla, M. B., et al. "Executive Function and Volume of the Basal Ganglia in Children with Tourette's Syndrome and Attention Deficit Hyperactivity Disorder," *Annals of Neurology,* v. 30, n. 3, Sept. 1991.

Fallon, Brian A. "What Is the Significance of Lyme Disease for Mental Health?" *Harvard Mental Health Letter,* Oct. 1, 1995, v.12, p. 8.

Faraone, S. V., et al. "A Family-Genetic Study of Girls with DSM III Attention Deficit Disorder," *American Journal of Psychiatry*, 1991. v. 148, pp. 112–117.

Giedd, J. N. "Quantitative Morphology of the Corpus Callosum in Attention Deficit Hyperactivity Disorder," *American Journal of Psychiatry*, 1994, v. 151, pp. 665–669.

Ginsburg, Benson E., et al., "A Genetic Taxonomy of Hyperkinesis in the Dog," *International Journal of Developmental Neuroscience*, v. 2, 1984, pp. 313–322.

Gladdwin, Mark T. et al. "Inappropriate Thyroid Gland Ablation in Patients with Generalized Resistance to Thyroid Hormone: A Common Sequel of a Rare Disorder," *Archives of General Medicine*, Jan. 8, 1996, v. 156, n. 1, p. 106 (4).

Gordon, Kevin, et al. "Valproic Acid Treatment of Learning Disorder and Severely Epileptiform EEG Without Clinical Seizures," *General Child Neurology*, 1996, v. 11, pp. 41–43.

Hartmann, T. *ADD Success Stories: A Guide to Fulfillment for Families with Attention Deficit Disorder.* (Grass Valley, Calif.: Underwood Books, 1995.)

Harvard Mental Health Letter, "Attention Deficit Disorder—Part I," April 1995, v. 11, n. 10, p. 1 (4).

Harvard Mental Health Letter, "Attention Deficit Disorder—Part II—Drug Therapy," May 1995, v. 11, n. 11, p. 1 (3).

Hauser, Peter, et al. "Attention Deficit-Hyperactivity Disorder in People with Generalized Resistance to Thyroid Hormone," *The New England Journal of Medicine*, April 8, 1993, v. 328, n. 14, p.997(5).

Health Legislation & Regulation, "H.R. 1797: Equitable Health Care for Neurobiological Disorders: Neurobiological Disorder Defined," Aug. 30, 1995.

Heiligenstein, Eric, and Keeling, Richard P. "Presentation of Unrecognized Attention Deficit Hyperactivity Disorder in College Students," *Journal of College Health*, v. 43, March 1995, pp. 226–228.

Henderson, Peter D. "Controls on ADHD Drugs Should be Reduced: (Editorial)," *American Pharmacy*, Sept. 1994, v. NS34, n. 9, p. 5.

Hendrick, Bill. "Study Suggests Attention Deficit Disorder Is Biological, Not Psychiatric," *Atlanta Constitution*, Nov. 16, 1995, p. B1.

Hyde, Thomas M. "Tourette's Syndrome: A Model Neuropsychiatric Disorder," *JAMA*, Feb. 8, 1995, v. 273, n. 6, p. 498 (4).

"Hyperactivity Disorder in Adults," *Patient Care*, Feb. 28, 1989, v. 23, n. 4, pp. 21–22.

Jankovic, J. "Deprenyl in Attention Deficit Associated with Tourette's Syndrome," *Archives of Neurology*, March 1993, v. 50, pp. 286–288.

Jansen, Peter S., et al. "Anxiety and Depressive Disorders in Attention Deficit Disorder with Hyperactivity: New Findings," *American Journal of Psychiatry*, Aug. 1993, v. 150, n. 8, p. 1203 (7).

Kashani, Javad et al. "Hyperactive Girls," *Journal of Operational Psychiatry*, v. 10, n. 2, 1979, pp. 145–148.

Kessler, Sheldon. "Drug Therapy in Attention Deficit Hyperactivity Disorder," *Southern Medical Journal*, v. 89, n. 1, Jan. 1996, pp. 33–38.

Kline, Rachel G. "The Role of Methylphenidate in Psychiatry," *Archives of General Psychiatry*, June 1995, v. 52, 429–433.

Kotwal, Dilnavaz, et al. "Computer Assisted Cognitive Training for ADHD: A Case Study Presented." Annual Convention of the American Psychological Association, Aug. 1994, Los Angeles.

Kwasman, Allen, et al. "Pediatricians' Knowledge and Attitudes and Knowledge Concerning Diagnosis and Treatment of Attention Deficit and Hyperactivity Disorders," *Archives of Pediatrics*, Nov. 1995, v. 149, n. 11, p. 1211 (6).

Lenckus, Dave. "Help on ADA Compliance Available to Employers," *Business Insurance*, Jan. 16, 1995, v. 29, 3, p. 43.

Lesaca, Timothy. "An Overview of Adulthood Attention Deficit Hyperactivity Disorder," *The West Virginia Medical Journal*, Nov. 1994, v. 90, pp. 472–474.

Lubar, J. F. "Discourse on the Development of EEG Diagnostics and Biofeedback for Attention Deficit/Hyperactivity Disorders," *Biofeedback and Self Regulation*, 1991, v. 16, pp. 200–225.

Lubar, Joel F., et al. "Evaluation of the Effectiveness of EEG Neurofeedback Training for ADHD in a Clinical Setting as Measured by Change in T.O.V.A. Scores, Behavioral Ratings and WISC-R Performance," *Biofeedback and Self Regulation*, 1995, v. 20, n. 1, pp. 83–99.

MacMullan, Jackie. "Fox Gets Attention," *Sports Illustrated,* March 4, 1996, v. 84, n. 9, p. 79.

Mann, C., et al. "Quantitative Analysis of EG Employees with Attention Deficit Hyperactivity Disorder: Controlled Study with Clinical Implications," *Pediatric Neurology,* v. 8, 1991, pp. 30–36.

Mannuzza, et al. "Adult Outcome of Hyperactive Boys," *Archives of General Psychiatry,* v. 50, 1993, pp. 565–576.

Matochik, John A., et al. "Cerebral Glucose Metabolism in Adult with Attention Deficit Hyperactivity Disorder after Chronic Stimulant Treatment," *American Journal of Psychiatry,* v. 151, n. 5, p. 658 (7).

Mayll, Mark. "Your Nutritional Essentials: Here Is a Guide to Using the 25 Most Important Mind Sharpening, Energy Increasing, Antiaging, Health Building Supplements to Achieve Your Mental, Physical Peak," *Natural Health,* March-April 1995, v. 26, n. 2, p. 85 (15).

McDonald, James J., et al. "Mental Disabilities Under the ADA: A Management Rights Approach," *Employee Relations Law Journal,* Spring 1995, v. 20, n. 4, p. 541 (29).

Milberger, S., et al. "Attention Deficit Hyperactivity Disorder and Co-Morbidity Disorders: Issues of Overlapping Symptoms," *American Journal of Psychiatry,* Dec. 1995, v. 152, n. 12, pp. 1793–99.

Miller, David, and Blum, Kenneth. *Overload: Attention Deficit Disorder and the Addictive Brain,* (Kansas City, Mo.: Andrews and McMeel, 1996.)

Mulholland, Thomas. "Human EEG Behavioral Stillness and Biofeedback," *International Journal of Psychophysiology,* v. 19, 1995, pp. 263–279.

Nadeau, Kathleen G., ed. *A Comprehensive Guide to Attention Deficit Disorder in Adults: Research, Diagnosis, and Treatment.* (New York: Brunner/Mazel, 1995.)

Nadeau, Kathleen G. *Survival Guide for College Students with ADD or LD.* (New York: Magination Press, 1994.)

Nahlik, James E. "New Thoughts on Attention-Deficit Hyperactivity Disorder," *Hospital Practice,* April 15, 1995, pp. 49–55.

National Institute of Mental Health. "Attention Deficit Hyperactivity Disorder." (Pamphlet) Sept. 1994, p. 1 (42).

Needleman, H. L. "Bone Lead Levels and Delinquent Behavior," *JAMA*, Feb. 7, 1996, v. 275 n. 5, p. 363 (7).

Power, Bruce. "Hyperactivity Grows Into Adult Problems," *Science News*, July 31, 1993, v. 144, n. 5, p. 70.

Ratey, John J. "Paying Attention to Attention in Adults." *CHADDer, A Publication by CH.A.D.D.*, Fall-Winter 1991, pp. 13–14.

Ratey, John J., et al. "Combination of Treatments for Attention Deficit Hyperactivity Disorder in Adults," *Journal of Nervous and Mental Disease*, v. 179, n. 11, Nov. 1991, pp. 699–701.

Ratey, John J., et al. "Special Diagnostic and Treatment Considerations in Women with Attention Deficit Disorder," in *A Comprehensive Guide to Attention Deficit Disorder in Adults*, Kathleen G. Nadeau, ed. (New York: Bruner/Mazel, 1995.)

Ratey, John J., et al. "Unrecognized Attention Deficit Hyperactivity Disorder in Adults Presenting for Outpatient Psychotherapy," *Journal of Child and Adolescent Psychopharmacology*, II 2, 267–275.

Reimherr, et al. "Cerebrospinal Fluid Homovanillic Acid and 5-Hydroxyindole Acetic Acid in Adults with Attention Deficit Disorder, Residual Type (ADD, RT)," *Psychiatry Research*, 1974, v. 11, pp. 71–78.

Riccio, Cynthia A., et al. "Neurological Basis of Attention Deficit Hyperactivity Disorder: Exceptional Children." Oct.-Nov. 1993, v. 60, n. 2, p. 118 (7).

Ritter, Malcolm. "Hyperactivity Gene." Associated Press, AP Newswire, 4-30-96 (Reference Lahouste, Gerald J., et al., April-May, *Journal of Molecular Psychiatry.*)

Robbins, Jim. "Wired for Miracles," *New Age Journal*, March-April 1996, pp. 94–1039.

Roeder, Jason. "Can Medication Change Behavior? (Treating Behavior Disorders in Autism with Medication)," *Exceptional Parent*, Nov. 1995, v. 25, n. 11, p. 50 (4).

Roizen, Nancy J, et al. "Psychiatric and Developmental Disorders in Families of Children with Attention Deficit Hyperactivity Disorder," *Archives of Pediatrics & Adolescent Medicine*, v. 150, n. 2, Feb 1996, p. 203(6a).

Rowe, K.S., et al. "Synthetic Food Coloring and Behavior: A Dose Response Effect in a Double Blind Placebo Controlled Repeated Measure Study," *Journal of Pediatrics*, 1994, v. 125, pp. 691–698.

Sacks, Oliver. *An Anthropologist on Mars.* (New York: Knopf, 1995.)

Schneider, Frank. "Self Regulation of Slow Cortical Potentials in Psychiatric Patients: Schizophrenia," *Biofeedback and Self Regulation*, v. 17, n. 4, 1992, pp. 277–292.

Schoenthaler, Stephen J. "Sugar and Children's Behavior [Editorial]," *New England Journal of Medicine*, v. 330, n. 26, June 30, 1994, pp. 1901–1904.

Schubiner, Howard, et al. "The Dual Diagnosis of Attention Deficit/Hyperactivity Disorder and Substance Abuse: Case Reports and Literature Review," *Journal of Clinical Psychiatry*, 1995, v. 56, pp. 146–150.

Schwadel, Francine. "Sears Sets Model for Compliance with Disabilities Act, Study Says," *Wall Street Journal*, March 4, 1995, p. B5.

Schweiger, Alice. "Not Just Kids," *Ann Arbor News*, July 14, 1993.

Searight, H. R. "Attention Deficit/Hyperactivity Disorder: Assessment, Diagnosis and Management," *General Family Practice*, March 1995, v. 40, n. 3, p. 270 (10).

Shaffer, David. "Attention Deficit Hyperactivity Disorder in Adults," *American Journal of Psychiatry*, May 1994, v. 151, n. 5, p. 663 (6).

Shaywitz, B. A., et al. "CSF Monoamine Metabolites in Children with Minimal Brain Dysfunction: Evidence for Alteration of Brain Dopamine," *Journal of Pediatrics*, 1977, v. 90, 76–71.

Shaywitz, S. E., and Shaywitz, B. A. "Attention Deficit Disorder: Current Perspectives," *Pediatric Neurology*, May-June 1987, v. 3, n.3, pp.129–135.

Sheki, W. "Residual Attention Deficit Disorder," *The Western Journal of Medicine*, Sept. 1989, v. 151, n. 3, p. 314.

Shekim, W. O., et al. "A Clinical and Demographic Profile of a Sample of Adults with Attention Deficit Hyperactivity Disorder, Residual State," *Comprehensive Psychiatric*, v. 31, n. 5, Sept.-Oct., 1990, pp. 416–425.

Sherman, Carl. "Venflaxine Offers an Alternative to Stimulants," *Clinical Psychiatry News*, July 1995, p. 5.

Sieg, K. G. "SPECT Brain Imaging Abnormalities in Attention Deficit Hyperactivity Disorder," *Clinical Nuclear Medicine,* Jan. 1995, v. 20, n. 1, pp. 55–60.

Spencer, T., et al. "ADHD and Thyroid Abnormalities: A Research Note," *Journal of Child Psychology and Psychiatry,* July 1995, v. 36, n. 5, pp. 879–885.

Spencer, Thomas, et al. "A Double Blind Crossover Comparison of Methylphenidate and Placebo in Adults with Childhood-Onset Attention Deficit Hyperactivity Disorder," *Archives of General Psychiatry,* June 1995, v. 52, p. 434 (10).

Steffgen, Kim A. "Check Compulsive Gamblers for Attention-Deficit Symptoms," *The Addiction Letter,* v. 11, n. 12, Dec. 1995, pp. 1–2.

Stein, Berhardt E. "Avoiding Drug Reactions: Seven Steps to Writing Safe Prescriptions," *Geriatrics,* Sept. 1994, v. 49, n. 9, pp. 28–35.

Stitch, Sally. "Why Can't Your Husband Sit Still?," *Ladies Home Journal,* Sept. 1993, v. 110, n. 9, p. 74 (2).

Stone, T. W., ed. *CNS Neurotransmitters and Neuromodulators; Dopamine.* (Boca Raton, Fla.: CRC Press, 1996.)

Stuart, Peggy. "Tracing Workplace Problems to Hidden Disorders," *Personnel Journal,* June 1992, v. 71, n. 6, p. 82(9).

Szpir, Michael. "Alcoholism, Personality and Dopamine," *American Scientist,* Sept.–Oct. 1995, v. 83, n. 5, p. 425 (2).

Taibbi, Robert. "Understanding ADHD: More than Just Active," *Current Health,* March 1995, v. 21, n. 7, p. 16 (2).

Tansey, Michael A. "Ten Year Stability of EEG Biofeedback Results for a Hyperactive Boy Who Failed 4th Grade Perceptually Impaired Class," *Biofeedback and Self Regulation,* v. 18, n. 1, 1993, 33–44.

Taylor, C. J. "Auditory and Visual Continuous Performance Test: A Comparison of Modalities," *ADHD/Hyperactivity Newsletter,* Fall–Winter 1994, n. 20.

TOVA; Greenberg, L. M. and Crosby, R. D. *Specificity and Sensitivity of the Test of Variables of Attention.* 1992.

Travis, John. "Imaging Hyperactive Brains," *Science News,* Nov. 25, 1995, v. 148, n. 22, p. 361.

Tzelepis, A., Schubner, H. and Warbasse, L. H. III. "Differential Diagnosis and Psychiatric Co-Morbidity Patterns in Adult Attention Deficit Disorder," in *A Comprehensive Guide to Attention Deficit Disorder in Adults. Research, Diagnosis and Treatment.* (New York: Brunner/Mazel, 1995.)

Wallace, A. E., et al. "Double Blind Placebo Controlled Trial of Methylphenidate in Older, Depressed, Medically Ill Patients," *American Journal of Psychiatry,* June 1995, v. 152, n. 6, p. 929 (3).

Ward, M. F., Wender, P. H., and Reimherr, F. W. "The Wender Utah Rating Scale: An Aid in the Retrospective Diagnosis of Childhood Attention Deficit Hyperactivity Disorder," *American Journal of Psychiatry,* v. 150, pp. 885–890.

Warren, Reed P., et al. "Is Decreased Blood Plasma Concentration of Complement C4B Protein Associated with Attention Deficit Hyperactivity Disorder?" *Psychiatry,* Aug. 1995, v. 34, n. 8, p. 1009 (6).

Weiss, Gabrielle. "Hyperactivity in Childhood [Editorial]," *New England Journal of Medicine,* Nov. 15, 1990, v. 323, n. 20, pp. 1413–1415.

Weiss, Gabrielle, and Hechtman, Lily Trokenberg. *Hyperactive Children Grown Up: ADHD in Children, Adolescents, and Adults.* (New York: Guilford Press, 1993.)

Weiss, Lynn. *Attention Deficit Disorder in Adults: Practical Help for Sufferers and Their Spouses.* (Dallas: Taylor, 1992.)

Wender, Paul H. *Attention Deficit Hyperactivity Disorder in Adults.* (New York: Oxford, 1995.)

Wender, Paul H., et al. "Bupruprion Treatment of Attention Deficit Hyperactivity Disorder in Adults," *American Journal of Psychiatry,* Aug. 1990, v. 147, n. 8, p. 1018 (3).

Wender, Paul H., et al. *The Hyperactive Child, Adolescent and Adult: Attention Deficit Disorder Through the Lifespan.* (New York: Oxford, 1987.)

Whiteman, T. A., and Novotni, Michele. *Adult ADD.* (Colorado Springs: Pinon Press, 1995.)

Wilens, M. D., et al. "A Systematic Assessment of Tricyclic Antidepressants in the Treatment of Adult Attention Deficit

Hyperactivity Disorder," *Journal of Nervous and Mental Disease,* v. 183, 1995, p. 48 (3).

Wilens, T. E., et al. "Pharmacotherapy of Adult Attention Deficit/Hyperactivity Disorder: Review," *General Clinical Psychopharmacology,* Aug. 1995, v. 15, pp. 270–79.

Wilens, T. E., M. D., et al. "Pharmacotherapy of Adult Attention Deficit/Hyperactivity Disorder: A Review," *Journal of Clinical Psychopharmacology,* v. 15, n. 4, Aug. 1995, pp. 270–279.

Wilkison, David. "Ritalin Warnings." Associated Press, March 27, 1996.

Williams, Laurie. "Understanding ADHD," *Essence,* July 1995, v. 26, n. 3, p. 102 (2).

Wolraich, Mark L., et al. "The Effect of Sugar on Behavior or Cognition in Children: A META Analysis," *JAMA,* Nov. 22, 1995, v. 274, n. 20, p. 1617 (5).

Wolraich, Mark L., et al. "The Effects of Diets High in Sucrose or Aspartame on the Behavior and Cognitive Performance of Children," *New England Journal of Medicine,* Feb. 3, 1994, v. 330, n. 5, pp. 301–307.

Zametkin, Alan J. "Attention-Deficit Disorder: Born to Be Hyperactive?" (Grand Rounds at the Clinical Center of the National Institutes of Health, *JAMA,* June 21, 1995, v. 273, n.23, p. 1871[4].

Zametkin, Alan J., et al. "Cerebral Glucose Metabolism in Adults with Hyperactivity of Childhood Onset." *New England Journal of Medicine,* 323: 1360–61 (20, 1413–1415).

Index

Also by Drs. Kandel and Sudderth

Spinal Tips: Physician's Home Remedy for Back or Neck Pain
Videotape, 46 minutes. $19.95 + $3.95 shipping and handling.

Chronic back and neck pain sufferers—you don't gain from pain! Get past the pain and enjoy your life again by following the expert, practical and immediately usable advice found in Spinal Tips. This video features simple exercises demonstrated by average people (not athletes or sports specialists) that will help you feel markedly better!

Relief from Hand and Arm Pain: Carpal Tunnel Syndrome and Repetitive Stress Injuries
Videotape, 16 minutes, $14.95 + $3.95 shipping and handling

Millions of people suffer from hand and wrist problems. If you are among them, this video can help greatly improve your problem or alleviate it altogether! Drs. Kandel and Sudderth offer important preventive measures and easy exercises you can integrate into your daily life. Also included are valuable descriptions and demonstrations of test doctors perform to detect repetitive stress injuries of the hand or wrist, as well as a discussion of surgical options.

Migraine—What Works!
Paperback, $12.95 + shipping and handling.

A comprehensive self-help book for managing migraine pain. Drs. Kandel and Sudderth offer expert counseling and review preventive measures and easy exercises to help avoid recurrent migraines.

Available from Prima Publishing.

Back Pain—What Works!
Paperback, $14.95 + shipping and handling.

A comprehensive self-help book for understanding the back and what individuals can do to cure, treat, and prevent back problems. Drs. Kandel and Sudderth address frequently asked questions concerning back pain as well as preventative measures and surgery.

Available from Prima Publishing.

Order from:
Pain Management Publishing
8380 Riverwalk Park Boulevard, Suite 320
Fort Myers, FL 33907

Or use your credit card and call 1-800-844-7880.

Visit Drs. Kandel and Sudderth on the Internet:
http://www.neurologist.com